# TEACHING AND ASSESSING IN NURSING PRACTICE

**Newer edition
available
Use with caution**

# The Authors

**Peter J Nicklin** MBA, MEd, DipEd(Lond), RGN, RMN, RNT
Having served as an officer in the Royal Army Medical Corps, Peter Nicklin entered the Health Service in 1983. NHS appointments have included Assistant Director of the North Lincolnshire School of Nursing, Director of the York and Scarborough College of Midwifery and Nursing and District Nurse Advisor for the York Health Authority. He has served as a committee member of the English National Board and is an executive member of the National Directors of Nurse Education Group. Peter Nicklin is a graduate of the Universities of London, Nottingham and Leeds; his MBA dissertation on 'the Quality of Nurse Education' received the inaugural *Yorkshire Post* award for Management Studies.

**Neil Kenworthy** MBA, BEd, RGN, RMN, RNT
Neil Kenworthy entered the NHS direct from secondary school and worked as a Nursing Assistant prior to becoming a student nurse. After 34 years, during which time he held posts of Principal Nursing Officer (Brentwood) and Director of Nurse Education (Lincoln), he left the NHS to work full-time as senior partner in a management and education consultancy company. He is a graduate of the Universities of Huddersfield and Leeds, and sustains his academic interests through working as an author and freelance editor.

# TEACHING AND ASSESSING IN NURSING PRACTICE

## An Experiential Approach

### Second Edition

**PETER J NICKLIN MBA MEd DipEd(Lond) RGN RMN RNT**

Director of Management and Corporate Services
and Director of Management Studies
North Yorkshire College of Health Studies

**NEIL KENWORTHY MBA BEd RGN RMN RNT**

Senior Partner, PNK Associates,
Education and Health Care Training Consultants, Lincoln

Foreword by
MAUREEN THEOBALD
Chairman, English National Board
London

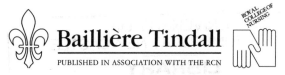

Baillière Tindall
PUBLISHED IN ASSOCIATION WITH THE RCN

London   Philadelphia   Toronto   Sydney   Tokyo

Baillière Tindall     24–28 Oval Road
London NW1 7DX

The Curtis Center
Independence Square West
Philadelphia, PA 19106–3399, USA

Harcourt Brace & Company
55 Horner Avenue
Toronto, Ontario M8Z 4X6, Canada

Harcourt Brace & Company, Australia
30–52 Smidmore Street
Marrickville
NSW 2204, Australia

Harcourt Brace & Company, Japan
Ichibancho Central Building
22-1 Ichibancho
Chiyoda-ku, Tokyo 102, Japan

© 1995 First published by Scutari Press
1996 Reprinted by Baillière Tindall and copyright transferred

This book is printed on acid-free paper

A catalogue record for this book is available from the British Library

ISBN 1-873853-20-3

Printed and bound in Great Britain by WBC Book Manufacturers Ltd, Bridgend, Mid Glamorgan.

# Contents

# Contributors

**John Dean** BA RGN CertEd RNT
Head of Professional & Vocational Studies, North Yorkshire College of Health
Studies

**Annette Lankshear** MA BSc RGN RHV RNT
Director of Research & Development, North Yorkshire College of Health
Studies

# Acknowledgements

The authors wish to convey their appreciation to John Dean and Annette Lankshear for their contributions to this edition and express their gratitude to Karen Barnes, Helen Garman and Anita Nicklin who have done all that incredibly difficult stuff that typically starts with 'Alt F . . .' and too frequently concludes with 'irretrievable disk error'!

**Note**   The term 'nurse' is used to simplify the presentation, but midwife or health visitor can be substituted in all cases.

# Foreword

I am delighted to have the opportunity to write a few words of welcome for the second edition of *Teaching and Assessing in Nursing Practice*. Its first edition proved to be very popular and this second edition is most timely.

No one is in any doubt that the years ahead are as likely to present as many challenges to nurses and nurse teachers as were presented in the past. But it is also true that together with these challenges will come increasing opportunities.

There is evidence all around of teachers grasping the opportunities made available to them, initiating changes of their own and bringing about improvements in learning opportunities and outcomes. Indeed, the contents of this new edition bear witness to the varied ways in which teachers of nursing in all settings continue to contribute to health care provision through education.

Readers of this book must take into account the implications of the conclusions contained in the Department of Health publication *The Challenges for Nursing and Midwifery in the 21st Century*. Similarly, nurses and nurse teachers are coming to terms with the implications of the UKCC's *Standards for Education and Practice*.

Such dynamic developments make the second edition of this popular aid to the thorny subject of teaching and assessment most welcome. It retains the essential ingredients of the first edition but now also contains additional chapters in order to meet changing needs. One such chapter concerns the issue of quality as a separate entity and pays proper recognition to total quality management. Now that we are working in a world of ever more specific contracts, measured outcomes and value for money, such a chapter will prove essential. Another is the developing theme of validation with attention to both professional and academic purpose. This second edition has its vision fixed on tomorrow.

With so many changes occurring in both courses and organisations, teachers can be forgiven for hoping that one day things will settle. We are forever challenged to remain up-to-date in all dimensions, be they clinical, research or education. This book will certainly aid us in the latter as all chapters have been revisited and are updated, with proper account being taken of the fact that students are currently assessed at both diploma and degree level. Likewise, for all of us who are involved in audit, the chapter on Recording and Reporting will be keenly sought.

Nurses are renowned for rising to meet demanding expectations, not least by their willingness to assess their own needs for further education and development. The potential to meet ever changing educational needs offered by the English National Board's Framework and Higher Award is increasingly being recognised by nurses at the cutting edge as they prepare themselves for the future. Teachers have responded with enthusiasm to this and every innovation.

The enthusiasm and energy shown by our professional colleagues merits the support such as is provided by this second edition of *Teaching and Assessing in Nursing Practice.* I wish it all the success it richly deserves.

MAUREEN THEOBALD
Chairman, English National Board

# Preface

The NHS has been subjected to so many changes in recent years that change seems too obvious to mention. But the very nature of change is changing. The notion that individuals and organisations move from one relatively stable state of affairs to a different but similarly stable state, through a transitional process called *change*, is entirely redundant in contemporary society. Change is not what it used to be, and the only safe prediction is that there are no safe predictions; this is the starting point for this second edition of *Teaching and Assessing in Nursing Practice*. The concluding comments in the first edition (1988) were concerned with the imminent implementation of Project 2000, which along with other strategic purposes, would ensure that nursing could attract sufficient young recruits from a declining labour market as the nation edged towards the 'demographic black hole'. The prophets proclaimed that whilst the previous decade had been about having no money (recession, inflation and so on), the next would be concerned with not having enough people (a balance of payments surplus, full employment, etc.) — 'there are no safe predictions'!

In this new world the motor for change is education and training. Successful organisations are characterised by being able to think of familiar things in different ways and employ people who can learn and learn anew. The authors well recall some years ago being described as 'perpetual students' — it was a term of derision. Whilst previously nurse registration might for some have been perceived as an end in itself, it is now self-evident that it is merely 'the end of the beginning' of career-long learning. Consequently, this book is intended to be a companion and guide for all those who have a responsibility for teaching and assessing whether their students are about to enter the profession or are in the autumn of their careers. Additionally the principles and skills described here are readily transferable to the teaching of patients and clients.

The book remains substantially based on the English National Board's 'Teaching and Assessing' (ENB 997 and 998) outline curricula. For this second edition the contents have been thoroughly revised, and there are new chapters on 'Quality in Teaching Practice' and 'Validation'. As in the previous edition the authors have attempted to balance theory with practice by applying the maxim that 'there is nothing as practical as good theory'.

PETER J NICKLIN
NEIL KENWORTHY
1995

# Preface to the First Edition

Amongst the large number of advances in nursing education during the past decade two stand out as being particularly significant: firstly, the rapid growth in the field of postbasic education, accompanied by the provision of increased resources and, secondly, the much heightened awareness of the need for the qualified nurse to receive adequate preparation for the teaching and assessing of students.

Many postbasic courses for registered nurses contain a teaching objectives element, particularly those concerned with 'developments in nursing'. Qualified nurses have received preparation for teaching and assessing in a number of ways: either informally through in-service training activities which may have included 'art of examining' courses or, more formally, through the very popular City and Guilds Further Education Teacher's Certificate course. Many nurses have received no preparation at all.

In writing this book the authors have sought to produce a resource for all those involved with the education and training of nurses in the practical setting; as a framework for the book the outline curriculum of the English National Board's Course 998 — Teaching and Assessing in Clinical Practice — has been used. A dilemma faced when designing the content of the book concerned the balance between theory and practice. Whilst not wanting to produce a 'workshop manual' on how to teach and assess, the authors were equally anxious not to end up with a book top heavy with theory and of very little practical value. Using the principle that 'there is nothing as practical as sound theory' the authors have endeavoured to provide a resource that will be of value to the 'knowledgeable doer' in preparation for the membership role. Their judgement is based upon personal experiences as teachers on both Further Education Teacher's Certificate (City and Guilds 730) and Certificate in Education courses, in addition to perceiving the needs of qualified nurses who are supervising students in the English National Board's pilot schemes in general nurse training. By adapting the experiential approach to teaching and learning described by Steinaker and Bell to nursing education and training, the authors believe that integration of theory with practice has a better chance of occurring — an educational principle which is so necessary in the practical setting. Not all nurses have a responsibility for the supervision of students, but there is an ever-increasing recognition of the nurse as an advocate, health adviser and health educator to patients, clients and relatives. The same obviously applies to those nurses who do carry out a teaching and assessing role with students. Perhaps this book therefore has a dual utility primarily to serve as a resource and guide to the qualified nurse in the mentorship role with students and, secondarily, to assist the nurse in fulfilling the broader role of health educator to all.

NEIL KENWORTHY
PETER J NICKLIN
1988

# 1
# Introducing the Experiential Approach

The vocational nature of nurse education has always required qualified nurses to act as supervisors and teachers to students. Whether those undertaking an educational programme are already registered and part of the NHS workforce or are students receiving bursaries, and supernumerary to the manpower equation, they will all require the mentorship of competent role models. It is clear that pre-registration education does not adequately equip nurses for a full teaching and assessing role, nor is it intended to do so. Without specific preparation the qualified nurse will be unable to undertake these functions competently, and this will deny students appropriate learning opportunities. Inevitably this in turn will have implications for the quality of care delivered to patients and clients.

Recognising the need to further improve standards of teaching and assessing, the English National Board (ENB) introduced its curriculum for 'Teaching and Assessing in Clinical Practice' (Course 998) in the mid 1980s, which has subsequently proved successful as an educational strategy and popular with course participants. This book is substantially based on the outline curricula of ENB 998 but its content and presentation are intended to have a practical application for all those involved in the teaching and assessing of health care programmes.

The major themes:

— the principles and practice of teaching, learning and assessing in clinical practice;
— the principles and practice of quality management in education, including evaluation and validation;
— creating a supportive learning environment;
— an introduction to counselling and counselling skills;

are discussed in the context of dynamic changes in health and education sector provision.

Believing these themes to be most relevant to the teaching and assessing function, the authors seek to present them in a way that is intended to guide the reader through the role by using an 'experiential' framework. This term is increasingly employed to describe a range of teaching and learning activities that have differing purposes and outcomes, and it can easily cause confusion, anxiety and even hostility. A word of caution is offered by Taylor (1983): 'Experiential learning is in danger of becoming yet one more educational fashion attracting a good deal of momentary attention, achieving a brief period of fashionable acceptance and little lasting acceptance'. In this text 'experiential' is used to describe a taxonomy devised and developed by Steinaker & Bell (1979). In recent years there has been an explosion of curriculum models and theories, each derived from a particular social, psychological and political stance. The 'experiential taxonomy' provides, in the authors' view, a potent framework for course design and delivery that can also supplement and strengthen other models. The taxonomy is suited to competence-based approaches to education and training such as National Vocational Qualifications (NVQ) where progressive levels of 'performance' criteria have to be identified, declared and measured.

Approximately 40 years ago educationalists attempting to identify and measure learning outcomes devised classifications of learning objectives. These classifications, or taxonomies, delineated the consequence of the educative process into three divisions or domains:

— The *cognitive* domain: the use of information and knowledge.
— The *affective* domain: attitudes, emotions and values.
— The *psychomotor* domain: doing and motor skills.

Some readers will be familiar with learning objectives set out in categories of *knowledge*, *skills* and *attitudes*. The problem with this form of classification is the tendency to examine thinking, feeling and doing in isolation rather than as a totally integrated activity. Although nursing is very much skill-based, nurses must avoid adopting those learning and teaching principles in which the acquisition of knowledge, skills and attitudes are seen as separate activities. The experiential taxonomy avoids this problem by providing a framework for understanding, planning and evaluating the meaning of total experiences. It not only describes the sequence of events (levels) that take the student from inability to achievement (Table 1.1) but offers appropriate learning objectives, learning principles, learning strategies, teaching strategies and assessment techniques.

Although the levels of the experiential taxonomy are further explored in later chapters on quality, learning, teaching and assessing, it is essential at this early stage to clarify not only what the experiential taxonomy is but also what it is not.

The terms 'experiential learning' and 'experiential taxonomy' must not be seen as synonymous. A curriculum can employ experiential learning techniques without being based upon an experiential taxonomy, and, similarly, courses built upon an experiential taxonomy will use learning strategies other

Table 1.1    Levels of the experiential taxonomy (after Steinaker & Bell 1979)

| 1 | Exposure level | The student is introduced to and is conscious of an experience |
|---|---|---|
| 2 | Participation level | The student has to make a decision to become part of the experience |
| 3 | Identification level | The student identifies with the experience both intellectually and emotionally |
| 4 | Internalisation level | The student progresses to this level when the experience begins to affect her or his life, changing behaviours and ways of doing things |
| 5 | Dissemination level | The student now expresses the experience, advocating it to others |

than, or in addition to, experiential methods. To many people experiential learning is characterised by role-playing, gaming and simulation and is employed predominantly in 'self-awareness' training. This is a very narrow interpretation of the approach and may even be considered a misconception by its advocates.

The experiential taxonomy is much more than a learning strategy: it comprises a series of stages through which the student progresses. These stages commence with the initial exposure to an experience and conclude with the incorporation of that experience into the student's observable behaviour. Experiences may be simulated or real, using role-play or placing the student in the patient setting. Listening to a formal lecture and reading a chapter in a textbook are experiences; both expose the student to new information, ideas and concepts, but proponents of experiential learning techniques would perhaps not recognise these activities as having a place in their approaches to learning.

A curriculum that has the experiential taxonomy as its framework will use a range of internally compatible teaching, learning and assessment strategies, each being complementary to, and supportive of, the others. Many of the strategies will reflect an experiential learning approach whilst others will be expository or teacher-centred. 'Internal compatibility' is probably the most significant feature of the taxonomy because it is not always easy to achieve. A close scrutiny of many curricula will reveal incompatibilities between the learning, teaching and assessment components of a course: a particular teaching strategy may be used because it happens to be fashionable yet is not compatible with the student's learning style, or assessment methods intended to measure learning outcomes are in reality only measuring a narrow band of cognitive skills.

The main purpose of this book is to examine some of the key principles and practical applications of the processes of teaching, learning, assessing and evaluating, yet it is necessary to explore a number of the associated factors that may influence these educational activities and even be a consequence of them. Changing patterns of care, a greater emphasis on applied research, new techniques and technologies, heightened consumer expectation, demands for increased efficiency and effectiveness and new management culture are significant features of contemporary health and social care provision. In this climate of change which Handy (1989) describes as 'discontinuous', such change is not predictable and requires new ways of thinking about familiar concepts. In such a climate, according to Handy, 'education has to become the single most important investment that any person can make in their own destiny'. This book which is cognisant of each professional's statutory obligation to maintain competence (UKCC 1994), aspires to encourage readers to assume a personal as well as professional responsibility for their learning and that of their students.

## References

Handy C (1989) *The Age of Unreason.* London: Hutchinson

Steinaker N & Bell R (1979) *The Experiential Taxonomy: A New Approach to Teaching and Learning.* New York: Academic Press

Taylor B (1983) *Experiential Learning.* Hatfield: NICEC Hatfield Polytechnic

UKCC (1994) *Standards for Education and Practice Following Registration.* London: UKCC

# 2
# Quality in Teaching Practice

The first edition of *Teaching and Assessing in Nursing Practice* (1988) devoted a single page to the issue of 'quality'. This second edition dedicates an entire chapter to the subject, accurately reflecting the logarithmic expansion of interest in quality and its increasing importance as an issue for the public sector in general and, in the context of this book, for health sector education in particular.

But what is quality? Can it be described or measured, and how, if at all, can the concept be applied to health sector education? When confronted by a similar question Ball (1985) declared:

> 'Quality in education is a subject extraordinarily difficult to come to grips with and full of pitfalls. There is no single final answer, and we should not look for it. But the issue cannot be avoided.'

This chapter will not provide a 'single final answer' but has the objective of defining quality, discussing the principles of the concept and their application to teaching and assessing in health sector education.

## The quality imperatives

Providers of health care and education would reasonably assert that, for them, quality has always been an issue of importance. However, much like the first edition of this book, quality was previously implied rather than explicit. During the past decade there has been mounting pressure for public sector services and the professionals they employ to give public and explicit account of the quality of the services they provide. Illustrative of these dynamically related pressures and imperatives are:

— political factors;
— socio-economic factors;
— admiration of the private sector.

## Political factors

Restraining public expenditure and obtaining value for money are central to the government's economic policies. Whereas previously the professions asserted and the public assumed 'quality as given', the 1970s saw a progressive loss of public confidence in a variety of professional groups, including those in health and education. Pollitt (1986) explains that 'perceived failures in public service programmes had shaken public confidence in professional competence, and left professional groups poorly placed to resist externally imposed tests of economy, competence and achievement'. Performance review was introduced to the NHS in 1983 with the publication of the DHSS Performance Indicators package. At a subsequent ministerial review, the ENB agreed that they would develop 'acceptable performance indicators for the purpose of monitoring the cost-effectiveness of nurse education'. In the same year Roy Griffiths (1983) conducted his enquiry into NHS management, claimed that differences between the private sector and the NHS were greatly overstated and concluded that the 'similarities between NHS management and business are more important . . . they are concerned with level of service (and) quality of product'. The government's pursuit of increased efficiency and improved quality was further reaffirmed in *Working for Patients* (Department of Health 1989). The creation of a managed market by making training the subject of contractual arrangements between purchasers and providers was considered necessary 'in order to . . . improve accountability for public funds . . . continue the drive for increased efficiency and effectiveness and greater value for money' (Department of Health 1989). As a consequence, in addition to the quality requirements of validators, providers must now meet the contracted quality specifications of their purchasers.

## Socio-economic factors

Social and economic changes have made customers more discerning. Improved material conditions, albeit not evenly distributed, have increased consumer choice and the expectations of the services they receive from both the private and public sectors. According to Corrigan *et al* (1988) 'wealth allows choice and thus comparisons . . . it is the enemy of blanket collective provision', concluding 'when there was not such wealth among the very large majority, collective provision for all its uniformity, brusqueness and remoteness, was not only tolerated but often welcomed'. As a consequence, public services had a tendency to see themselves as providing services *to* the public rather than *for* the public, frequently assuming that they 'knew what was best for the customer' rather than focusing on the customer's actual needs. The emergence of consumerism has challenged and significantly changed the nature and style of many public services, including health and education. The rights of consumers feature prominently in the policies of both main political parties. A Labour government would establish a Quality Commission to promote the quality of health and education and require service providers to publicise their standards. In 1991 the government published *The Citizen's*

*Charter,* which requires public service providers to publish explicit standards and demands that 'services should be run to suit the convenience of customers, not staff'. Of particular importance to health sector education is *The Charter for Higher Education* (Department of Education 1993).

### Admiration of the private sector

The relative success of economic policy and growth of confidence in the private sector during the early 80s has been offered as an argument for the government's concern that higher education and the NHS should become more 'businesslike' and quality conscious. The achievements of former public sector organisations such as British Airways and British Telecom resulted in an admiration of private sector practices. Compulsory competitive tendering has not only brought public sector services into direct operational contact with the private sector but also encouraged 'in-house' or direct labour services to scrutinise the cost and quality of their provision in a way that was perceived as unnecessary in a non-competitive environment. In recent years there has been a substantial increase in 'cross sector flows' of not only services but also personnel. As the boundaries between the two sectors become increasingly permeable, the skills and attitudes of the private sector are having a significant influence on the delivery of health sector education.

These 'quality imperatives' have resulted in a fundamental change in the focus of public sector services. When applied to health sector education, these can be summarised as illustrated in Fig. 2.1.

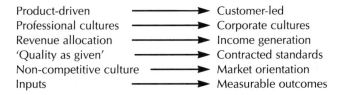

Product-driven ⟶ Customer-led
Professional cultures ⟶ Corporate cultures
Revenue allocation ⟶ Income generation
'Quality as given' ⟶ Contracted standards
Non-competitive culture ⟶ Market orientation
Inputs ⟶ Measurable outcomes

Fig. 2.1    Quality imperatives

There can be little doubt that political and socio-economic changes have conspired to create a market in health sector education. As this market becomes increasingly competitive the pressure for educational providers to demonstrate the quality of their services and products intensifies. The introduction of Working Paper 10 contracts, with their attendant quality specifications and the intense competition for a declining pre-registration market, has concentrated the thinking of educationalists on quality as the key to contract acquisition. Whilst previously quality may have been perceived as 'fashionable' but not essential, and Dr W Edwards-Deming's cannon — 'survival is not compulsory' — regarded as TQM (total quality management) speak, there can be few engaged in the business of health sector education who fail to recognise that quality is no longer a soft concept but a hard construct — the arbiter of survival.

The preceding paragraphs have described the pressures and incentives for quality improvement and have been concerned with 'Why quality?' But what is quality? As previously noted it is an elusive concept 'and full of pitfalls'. In the subsequent sections of this chapter, an attempt will be made to define and describe the principles of quality in the context of health sector education.

## Quality principles

Quality is a notoriously difficult concept to come to grips with. Definitions include:

— grade of goodness;
— fitness for purpose;
— degree of excellence;
— conformance not elegance;
— zero defects;
— right first time;

and many more. Shaw (1986), when confronted with this potentially bewildering list, suggested that 'watertight definitions of "quality" and related words are too elusive to merit the time of practical people. But some common ground is essential'. Subsequently the ENB (1993) has 'attempted to demystify these complexities' by identifying the principles which underpin quality in nurse education. According to the ENB quality is:

— well related to the purpose and functions of the institution, departments and teams, and to the corporate objectives of the service providers/ purchasers and regions;
— a cultural process reflecting the values and views of all those who invest in and are recipients of nursing and midwifery education; for example students, service colleagues, resource providers, professional colleagues, patients and clients;
— related to the achievement of economy, efficiency and effectiveness, particularly the latter;
— a journey, not a destination, and a process that is cyclical, continuous, systematic, permanent and regular and that demonstrates continuous institution improvement and development;
— a process that is responsive to consumer and customer needs and identifies student satisfaction;
— a process that involves professionals engaging in reflective deliberation and critical reflection on practice;
— a programme characterised by leadership and managerial commitment that demonstrates grass roots ownership;
— a democratic, participative process that is everybody's responsibility;
— a programme that is responsive to the political agenda of the time, for example the requirements of the White Paper, *Working for Patients*, Working Paper 10.

The dominant theme of these principles is a concern for the customer, so consequently a practical definition of quality might be:

meeting or exceeding the comprehensively understood needs of customers.

## Customers and consumers

It has been the convention to describe the users of public sector services as consumers rather than customers, the term 'customer' implying direct payment for a commodity or service. This differentiation is not merely semantic but attitudinal and a potential barrier to quality. For some there is the notion that 'consumers' are not paying, indeed receiving their service free. As there is no cash transaction between recipient and provider, both participants may be inclined to accept indifferent quality, although there is no such inclination when a provider is confronted by a 'customer' with a cheque book. Consequently in the course of this discussion, the terms customer and consumer are synonymous. Nicklin and Lankshear (1990) identify five customers of nurse education:

—  The public.
—  Academic and validating bodies.
—  Commissioning agents (employers).
—  Students.
—  Staff of the college.

These customers all receive or exchange services with the college. If quality is about meeting customer or consumer needs, what are these? Martin Smith (1986) proposes five 'tenets of consumerism', principles which can be usefully applied to health sector education:

—  *Access:* the ease of obtaining services. This embraces many issues but is essentially concerned with the elimination of discriminatory practices that deny customers equitable access to services. This may relate to geographical location, hours of opening, the provision of facilities for the disabled, crèche facilities and recruitment and selection practices.
—  *Choice:* assumes unrestricted access, but access to what? Customers need to influence the range and style of services they use. This can be achieved through marketing surveys, 'user groups', course development teams, course evaluations, staff consultative committees and satisfaction surveys.
—  *Information:* the availability of timely and accurate information is clearly linked to choice, and a range of techniques and technologies is required. These include the college prospectus, annual report, newsletters, curriculum documents and team briefings.
—  *Redress:* the Citizen's Charter requires that 'when things go wrong there must be a swift and simple way of putting them right'. Colleges must provide an effective complaints system that, in addition to providing redress, will enable services to be improved.

— *Representation:* the interests of customers should be represented at all levels throughout the college. Some would argue that the NHS reforms have reduced public representation, with non-executive board members being appointees rather than elected representatives. There remains, however, considerable scope for customer representation in the provision of health sector education. Customers should be represented throughout a college's committee structure. In addition to those previously described, validating panels, examination boards, student councils and ethics committees are illustrative of opportunities for customer participation and representation.

## Staff as customers

Above, five groups of customers of nurse education were identified. Employers purchase skills or research expertise for the delivery of patient care, students receive a service in the form of education and training, the public are potential recruits or clients of the health service and validators exchange services with the college. For some the notion of employees as customers is a novel if not surprising concept. Regarding staff as *internal customers* and adopting the philosophy of *internal marketing* is fundamental to service quality. According to Lewis (1988) 'personnel are seen as the first market of a service company and the objective of internal marketing is to get motivated and customer-conscious staff'. Internal marketing has two related strands:

— Employees receive explicit cues from management on their attitudes and values. If staff are treated with respect and concern and are afforded courtesy and regard, these values will in turn be transmitted to the external customer. It is salutory to note that the converse is also true. In the words of Clemmer (1990) 'it defies logic to expect exceptional behaviour from people who are not treated exceptionally'.
— Employees within a service organisation provide and receive services through an internal service chain. For example, the recruitment process may commence with a telephone inquiry, details are passed to another employee who despatches a prospectus and application form, which is subsequently returned and passed for a decision to a course manager, and so on . . . until the student successfully accesses the course of study. The staff involved and the broad range of skills applied can be described as a 'quality chain' (Fig. 2.2). Each participant in the chain receives work (customer), applies skills, processes the work and passes it on (supplier) to the next stage. If at any stage the work done is flawed, it will have to be returned to the supplier and reworked, hence Crosby's (1978) maxim 'Quality is free'. In his view, there is no such thing as the economics of quality — it is always cheaper to do the job right first time. Indeed it is estimated that correction of mistakes can represent as much as 40% of the operating cost of service industries. That says nothing of the costs of failure: the frustration, anger, blame, loss of esteem and ultimately the loss of a customer.

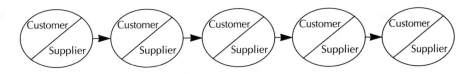

Fig. 2.2    Quality chain

Explicit concern for the needs of customers (internal and external), the prevention of failure and the quest for continuous improvement are features of a quality service and fundamental to total quality management.

## Total quality management

Total quality management (TQM) is the strategic approach to providing the best possible services and products. Subordinate to TQM are quality assurance, quality control and inspection procedures (Fig. 2.3).

The concepts of inspection, quality control and quality assurance are well understood in health sector education. Checking for errors during and after a process is common practice and applies to administration and academic procedures. The use of statistics (performance indicators), evaluations, placement and educational audit, operational standards, satisfaction surveys and validation are evident in all colleges. TQM pervades all functions and is concerned with attitudes and the culture of the organisation. Hallawell (1993) describes the benefits of TQM when applied to a college of nursing and midwifery; it:

— increases job satisfaction;
— decreases extra work through reduction of errors;
— enables people to work 'smarter' not 'harder';
— encourages positive working relationships;
— increases the skill portfolio of all staff;
— encourages innovative practice;
— makes it 'safe' to get it wrong when attempting improvement;
— encourages supportive people management;
— involves all staff in the development of the college;
— gives recognition to the contribution of all staff.

Fundamental to the successful implementation of TQM are leadership and empowerment. Wash (1991) asserts that 'Total Quality Management is more than tools, techniques, process and structures . . . [it's about] managerial behaviour, skills and style of leadership . . . managers need to understand the links between quality processes and their behaviour and skills'. He identifies the following quality leadership behaviours; a leader:

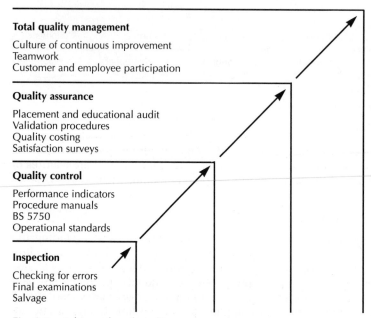

**Total quality management**

Culture of continuous improvement
Teamwork
Customer and employee participation

**Quality assurance**

Placement and educational audit
Validation procedures
Quality costing
Satisfaction surveys

**Quality control**

Performance indicators
Procedure manuals
BS 5750
Operational standards

**Inspection**

Checking for errors
Final examinations
Salvage

Fig. 2.3    A hierarchy of quality management

— gets full use out of staff, knows their capabilities, encourages, considers their feelings and aspirations;
— has strength of purpose, is willing to deal with important issues head-on, no matter how tough;
— does the job for the company and the customer, puts in 110%, sees self as part of the team;
— is open and honest, approachable and dependable, a good listener, and displays an interest in other points of view;
— will take action, 'let's go for it';
— will discuss decisions and listen to arguments, disseminates all relevant information;
— inspires confidence and is to be trusted — decisions have been reached and thought through;
— delegates — demonstrates trust and encourages ownership;
— asks for people's ideas — is prepared to be persuaded by logical, relevant discussion;
— cares about people and their problems, is interested on a personal level;
— gives realistic objectives, has clear criteria and ground rules;
— knows what is going on, has a bigger picture, looks at problems globally and can communicate the company view.

Whilst managers have subordinates, leaders have followers. Managers tell people what to do, whilst leaders empower their people. 'Empowerment' has contemporary currency in the language of management and education, and is fundamental to TQM. Peters (1987) claims that 'the most effective leaders, political or corporate, empower others to act . . . powerful leaders make followers more powerful in pursuit of a commonly held dream, jointly defined'. Empowerment is not merely a loosening of the managerial reins; it has three distinctive elements.

— *Capability:* implies that employees have the appropriate knowledge, skills and attitudes competently to exercise their role. Organisations such as colleges are dynamic, so role specifications require to be reviewed frequently and skills deficits addressed through a system of performance review and personal development planning. The training needs of administrative and clerical staff are particularly important but too frequently neglected. 'Front of house' staff are the shop window of the organisation. The promptly answered telephone and the courteous well-informed secretary are as essential to a college's viability as is the quality of its teaching.
— *Confidence:* to act without reference to a superior, to innovate and take informed risks is essential in providing a quality service. Employees need to work in a climate of trust, in a culture that is more concerned with 'catching someone doing something right' than apportioning blame for errors. Although quality is about 'getting it right first time', quality organisations can tolerate mistakes, can learn from them and move on. Delegation is the *sine qua non* of empowerment and is characterised by managers who 'let go' and grant to their staff autonomy that is real and significant.
— *Congruence:* or 'alignment' is the third element of empowerment. Staff of the college may be highly skilled and have considerable autonomy but still not be empowered. Empowerment is about 'doing the right thing' as well as 'doing things right'. Empowered staff are aligned to their college's mission and corporate objectives and have equal clarity about their role and contribution to their achievement. To be aligned, staff need to be involved and engaged in the development of strategy and policy and be informed of changes in practice or procedure.

## Total ethical management

The preceding sections of this chapter have described the principles and benefits of TQM. Implementing TQM is however notoriously difficult, and it is estimated that 60% of organisations fail in the attempt. Kinston (1992) offers a compelling explanation. TQM is a 'value system' and although organisations may be experienced in changing their methods and operations, few are experienced or competent in changing or managing values. In the words of Kinston, 'values are currently being handled in the typical firm about as effectively as quality was in the 1950's . . . the time has come for those who lead organisations to give more attention to the way values affect results'. Kinston has developed the concept of total ethical management (TEM), its ten core principles providing the context for TQM and making its successful implementation more likely. TEM is about the effective and deliberate management of values enhancing not only the organisation's performance but also its reputation.

## A quality taxonomy

Crosby (1978) describes five stages of quality management maturity, a continuum that embraces the recognition by management that 'quality' has organisational benefits, and proceeds to a final stage when quality management is considered vital to the organisation. When the experiential taxonomy (Steinaker & Bell 1979) is applied to quality, it provides a comprehensive framework for auditing an organisation's progress towards implementing TQM. A quality taxonomy involves:

1  *Exposure.* The college is introduced to the concept of quality through intrinsic motivation and extrinsic pressures.
2  *Participation.* The college commits time and resources to developing a strategy for quality improvement. Management and staff are trained in principles and techniques.
3  *Identification.* The college implements its strategy, its customers (internal and external) becoming committed to developing techniques and procedures to enhance quality.
4  *Internalisation.* The college's characteristic style of doing things is dominated by a concern for quality. Quality principles are adapted and applied in new settings.
5  *Dissemination.* The college seeks to influence others and commends its approach as imperative to customers.

## Quality in practice

So far this chapter has concerned itself with the quality imperative — the why — and the principles of quality — the what; it now turns its attention to quality in practice — the how. As suggested earlier quality is not a new phenomenon, and it is worth identifying the quality-related procedures that are currently applied to health sector and higher education. Peer review resides at the heart of academic and professional quality systems. Validation procedures have been and will remain the cornerstone of educational quality and are fully discussed in Chapter 11.

Whilst peer review will retain its central role in assuring the quality of education, it has in itself proven insufficient to meet externally imposed demands. During the 1980s 'quality' became synonymous with 'performance' and 'performance indicators'. Pollitt (1986) explains that performance is a seductive concept — 'it exudes an aroma of dynamism and purposeful effort. It suggests a sorting out of the good from bad' — and in these terms it can be constructed as a non-technical, non-political, objective and neutral indicator of quality. In 1987 the Royal College of Nursing (RCN) developed performance indicators for nurse education, and two years later the ENB published *A Guide to Assessing Performance and Quality in Nursing and Midwife Training Institutions* (ENB 1989), which included a proposed set of performance indicators. The ENB acknowledged the tenuous link between inputs and outcomes and cautioned against the use of performance indicators (PIs) as a proxy for quality, concluding, 'performance indicators . . . have no reliable meaning unless there is some parallel process which guarantees standards'. There is undeniably a tension between notions of performance that give pre-eminence to efficiency (lowest cost) and scant regard to other dimensions of quality such as appropriateness and acceptability. The rate and volume of fruit passing through the supermarket check out (PIs) yield little information on its freshness or complaints received. Similarly recruitment, attrition, pass rates and financial ratios are useful indices of the college's performance but say little about the student experience, the amenities of the college, employers' satisfaction with the skills taught or the morale of the teaching staff. Standards are fundamental to quality; the NHSME (1993) requires that all NHS authorities specify and continuously review standards of service. According to Nicklin and Lankshear (1990) 'standards can be measured. Standards are qualitative and quantitative measures by which nurse education can be judged and compared'.

## Standards

The literature of nursing and education is replete with models and theories of standard setting, all of which contain four key characteristics. They must be:

— *Meaningful.* Standards need to be owned and acceptable. Some standards are derived from statute or regulations whilst others are locally generated. All those with a legitimate interest in the standard of a service should contribute to setting standards. Standards need to be agreed or at least understood as imposition merely invites rejection. Meaningful also implies achievable; there is little value in setting standards that cannot be resourced. This does not preclude changing techniques and practices, which may simultaneously release resources and improve performance.
— *Measurable.* Standards should be contiguous to the college's mission and values and be written in terms of observable phenomenon. Together with conditions under which achievement is expected, standard setting also requires a 'measured' approach. Standards need to be memorable, which means not too many. In any department there are probably between eight and ten key standards that everybody knows and wishes to be judged by.
— *Monitored.* Standards require to be monitored for compliance and variance. This may be the random sampling of the frequency with which correspondence has been answered or scripts marked and returned, against an agreed standard. Monitoring may require technology and also

committed staff who are skilled in asking the right questions and who are prepared to receive and respond to complaints. It is also the mechanism by which the organisation catches somebody doing something right!

— *Managed.* The entire process of setting and achieving standards has to be managed. A framework for establishing and auditing standards will be considered shortly, but in addition staff need to be trained to use standards and may require training to achieve them. Consequently individual performance review and personal development planning contribute significantly to setting and achieving standards.

Employing these four key characteristics of standard setting, standards can be framed as indicated in Fig. 2.4.

Whilst most people find little to disagree with on the principles of quality, getting to grips with quality and doing something practical can certainly be elusive, hence Pirsig's (1974) somewhat despairing observation 'so round and round you go, spinning mental wheels, and nowhere finding any place to get traction'. If the principles of quality are to be mobilised, an operational framework is required. Educational audit provides a framework for the systematic and critical analysis of educational standards, embracing both qualitative and illuminative evidence. It seeks to determine whether planned arrangements are appropriate and implemented effectively to achieve the college's objectives. The four stages of audit are illustrated in Fig. 2.5.

| A | **AREA**   Communications | | |
|-----|-----------------------------|---|---|
| 1.0 | **OBJECTIVE**   To provide courteous, timely and accurate information | | |
| S | **Standard** | **Monitoring criteria** | **Management reponsibility** |
| 1.1 | Complaints to receive written acknowledgement within 4 days and full explanation within 14 days. | Complaints and appreciations register to be checked by Vice Principal each week. Submit register to College Board each quarter. | Policy formulation. Staff development and training. Director of Personnel |
| 1.2 | All 'routine' correspondence to receive acknowledgement or reply within 5 working days. | Compare receipt/reply dates and content of randomly selected correspondence monthly. | Provide feedback on compliance. Customer Services Manager |

Fig. 2.4   Specimen standards

In recent years a myriad of informants on educational audit have emerged, for example:

— British Standards Institute (BS 5750);
— Citizen's Charter (Charter for Higher Education; Department for Education 1993);
— Citizen's Charter (Patient's Charter);
— Higher Education Quality Control (Audit Methods and Procedures);
— Further Education Unit (Educational Audit);
— ENB (Guidelines for Educational Audit, 1993);
— NHSME (Framework of Audit for Nursing Services, 1991).

The ENB (1993) has issued guidelines on educational audit to assist colleges in preparing annual reports and quinquennial reviews. The Board's guidance is not intended to be 'prescriptive or restrictive' but seeks to disseminate examples of good practice. The ENB's framework for audit is an adaptation of the NHSME's (1991) *Framework of Audit for Nursing Services.* The QualCube framework (Nicklin & Lankshear 1994) described here is a refinement of the authors' earlier work and has cognisance of the approach advocated by the ENB and NHSME.

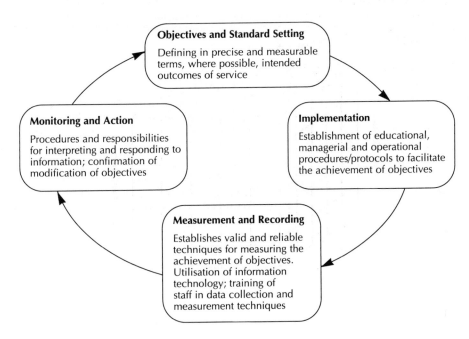

**Objectives and Standard Setting**

Defining in precise and measurable terms, where possible, intended outcomes of service

**Monitoring and Action**

Procedures and responsibilities for interpreting and responding to information; confirmation of modification of objectives

**Implementation**

Establishment of educational, managerial and operational procedures/protocols to facilitate the achievement of objectives

**Measurement and Recording**

Establishes valid and reliable techniques for measuring the achievement of objectives. Utilisation of information technology; training of staff in data collection and measurement techniques

Fig. 2.5    Education audit cycle

## Educational audit — QualCube

QualCube (Fig. 2.6) has been constructed to provide a systematic and dynamic framework for setting standards, appraising activity and generating quality improvements that are consistent with a college's explicit values. The model has three dimensions:

— *Business elements:* the core functions of the college.
— *Audit characteristics:* dimensions of educational quality.
— *Audit customers:* internal and external customers.

Each of these three dimensions has five subdivisions, enabling the organisation to be interrogated or audited in 125 activity cells (5 × 5 × 5). These cells are neither equal nor finite, and it is evident that some cells merit more extensive enquiry than others. In practical terms no audit can aspire to investigate in depth much more than the most important quality procedures, structures and mechanisms.

*Business elements*

**Leadership, management and administration**   A fundamental principle of TQM is the need for staff alignment with the organisation's vision. Thus the clarity and ownership of mission, values and purposes become a key indicator of quality. Consequently managerial, financial and communication structures must be examined, as must administrative and support systems.

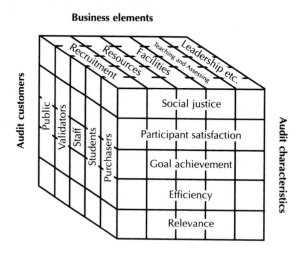

Fig 2.6    QualCube educational audit framework (Nicklin & Lankshear, 1994)

**Teaching and assessing (theory and practice)**    This includes such features as the integrity and consistency of curriculum design, the imparting of knowledge and skills and the fostering of attitudes. The qualifications, qualities and abilities of teaching and clinical staff are examined as is the degree of validity and reliability of adopted assessment strategies. Within client care areas, clinical credibility and the research basis of care must be considered.

**Facilities**    This category covers the suitability of buildings, fittings and furnishings, together with classroom, social and residential accommodation, but excludes clinical placements.

**Educational resources**    This includes library, media resource, laboratory and technical facilities.

**Recruitment**    Recruitment encompasses the process of attracting, processing and selecting students.

*Audit characteristics*

**Social justice**    This item comprises the mechanisms for ensuring fairness, equity, even-handedness and antidiscriminatory practice. Compliance with policies and operational procedures that ensure social and physical accessibility and availability is tested.

**Participant satisfaction**    This examines the extent to which the needs of customers are explicitly understood and the degree to which they find the products and services acceptable.

**Goal achievement**    This explores the effectiveness of the organisation — the extent to which the college achieves intended aims and has marketing strategies that generate services and products that demonstrate fitness for purpose.

**Efficiency**    Efficiency is concerned with the ratio of inputs to outputs and is in effect concerned with the cost-effective utilisation of resources and the elimination of waste.

**Relevance**    This requires that the development of products and services meets contemporary health and social care requirements based upon sound market intelligence and research.

*Customers*

**Public**    This category is comprised of the lay population of the college's catchment area whose interests are represented and protected by the non-executive members of the college management board.

**Validators**    These include the academic and vocational institutions and professional bodies that confer academic, vocational or professional validity on the college's programmes.

**Staff of the college**    This facet demands that the college demonstrates the principle of internal marketing, regarding staff as 'internal customers'.

**Students**    Included within this category are those customers who register with the college to undertake a programme of study.

**Purchasers**    This group is distinguished by its capacity to purchase the products or services of the college on behalf of itself or others.

The utility of the QualCube approach resides in its three-dimensional and dynamic construction. For example, producing standards or eliciting PIs relating to efficiency and teaching from a purchaser's perspective might suggest that the teacher:student ratio be reduced so as to constrain the unit cost of training. This may be at variance with teaching and participant satisfaction from a student perspective and so on — 'There is no single final answer' (Ball 1985) — but the skill of managing quality lies in recognising these inevitable tensions and making considered judgements in providing acceptable solutions. A multidimensional approach increases focus, definition and precision when used in the context of audit. As in navigation the greater the number of reference points, the more accurate the orientation. Such a framework can be employed to develop:

— performance indicators;
— financial indicators;
— student satisfaction surveys;
— teaching audit tools;
— clinical placement audits;
— first destination employer surveys;
— leadership surveys;

and other instruments. The strength of applying a single model or framework in the construction of audit instruments or performance indicators is that theoretical assumptions and values are held as a constant. Consequently results are inclined to be more reliable than if techniques and instruments from different origins are employed.

In this chapter the author has attempted to introduce the principles of quality and apply them to health sector education. Any observer or commentator on quality has an overwhelming choice of references as the subject of quality has spawned a disproportionate number of gurus who have, in turn, generated a plethora of inspiring 'sound bites'.

The literature frequently refers to quality as an 'unending journey' but it should be remembered the route lies in the familiar landscape of daily college life. As Gorman observes:

'A lot of people have fancy things to say about quality including me, but it's just a day in day out, ongoing, never ending, unremitting, persevering, compassionate type of activity.'

## References

Ball C (1985) *Fitness for Purpose*. Guildford: NFER-Nelson

Clemmer J (1990) *Firing on all Cylinders*. London: Piatkus

Corrigan J *et al* (1988) *Socialism, Merit and Efficiency*. Fabian Society Pamphlet No. 530. London: Fabian Society

Crosby P B (1978) *Quality is Free*. Maidenhead: McGraw-Hill

Department for Education (1993) *The Charter for Higher Education*. London: HMSO

Department of Health (1989) *Working for Patients*. Working Paper No 10. London: HMSO

English National Board (1989) *Figuring out Performance*. London: ENB

English National Board (1993) *Guidelines for Educational Audit*. London: ENB

Griffiths R (1983) *NHS Management Enquiry*. London: HMSO

Hallawell R (1993) Quality management in a college of nursing and midwifery. *British Journal of Nursing*, **2**:13

HM Government (1991) *The Citizen's Charter*. London: HMSO

Kenworthy N & Nicklin P (1988) *Teaching and Assessing in Nursing Practice*. London: Scutari Press

Kinston W (1992) *Working with Values for Results*. London: Sigma

Lewis B (1988) Customer care in service organisations. *International Journal of Health Care Quality Assurance*, **2**:1

NHSME (1991) *Framework of Audit for Nursing Services*. London: DoH

NHSME (1993) *Planning Guidelines 1994/95*. London: DoH

Nicklin P J & Lankshear A J (1990) Quality matters. *Nursing Times*, **86**:31

Nicklin P J & Lankshear A J (1994) *The Cube Route to Quality*. Unpublished research project; North Yorkshire College of Health Studies

Peters T (1988) *Thriving on Chaos*. London: Pan

Pirsig R M (1974) *Zen and the Art of Motorcycle Maintenance*. London: The Bodley Head

Pollitt C (1986) Beyond the management model. *Financial Accountability and Management*, **2**:3

Shaw C D (1986) *Introducing Quality Assurance*. Project Paper 64. London: King's Fund.

Smith M (1986) *The Consumer Case for Socialism*. Fabian Society Pamphlet No 513. London: Fabian Society

Steinaker N & Bell R (1979) *The Experiential Taxonomy*. New York: Academic Press

Wash M (1991) Quality through leadership. *Managing Service Quality*, **1**:2

# 3
# The Principles of Learning

## Introduction

All education programmes for nurses, midwives and health visitors at pre-qualifying level, and many at post-qualifying level, represent attempts to resolve the age old questions:

— How much time should be spent learning in the practice setting, compared with the classroom or laboratory?
— Which things are best learned in the practice setting and which in the classroom or laboratory?

Arguments around these issues are passionately conducted, with various factions arguing furiously for more time to be spent in close proximity to patients and practising health professionals whilst others argue for more emphasis on underlying theories and principles.

However the arguments proceed, there is no doubt that learning opportunities in practice settings continue to be of fundamental importance in the preparation and continuing education of practitioners. As the UKCC (1986) states:

> 'Placements are essential and should be planned systematically so that theory can be applied critically by students — such placements [should be] planned solely to meet educational needs.'

This statement, made with reference to Project 2000, not only illustrates the importance of spending time in practice settings but also emphasises the purpose of placement time for students. As a principle for good practice the UKCC statement has an application wider than just pre-registration nursing education programmes.

It is the learning that takes place outside of the classroom and within the patient and client care environment that forms the subject for consideration in this chapter. Rather than dwell upon dictionary meanings of the term 'learning' or the many definitions offered by writers on the subject of education, the definition offered by Curzon (1990) is perhaps a useful benchmark, particularly where learning is taking place in a practical setting. Curzon considers learning as the:

'Apparent modification of a person's behaviour through his activities and experiences so that his knowledge, skills and attitudes, including models of adjustment towards his environment, are changed, more or less permanently.'

What does this mean when applied to students and their anticipated or required learning in a practical experience placement? It usually means the acquisition of the stated objectives commonly expressed in the form of the cognitive, effective and psychomotor taxonomies, i.e. Bloom (1964), Krathwohl et al (1968) and Simpson (1966). The separation of knowledge, attitudes and physical skills is convenient when designing learning objectives but is it realistic? Do students learn chunks of knowledge in isolation from having a feeling towards the subject, and are physical skills acquired in the absence of any knowledge? Whilst advocating Curzon's definition of learning as a practical proposition for nurse education, it can probably be modified somewhat to remove the artificiality of the three domains of knowledge, skills, attitudes. The description of learning as applied to nurse education in the practice setting would now read:

'the measurable effect of the sum total of the planned and unplanned experiences upon the student, in both quantitative and qualitative terms.'

How these responses to experience are measured will form the subject of a separate chapter. It is appropriate at this stage to refer briefly to some of the more important theories of learning so that practice-based teachers can make the best use of the learning opportunities as they arise or are engineered within their care environment.

## Learning theories

Learning theories provide frameworks for studying the processes associated with learning. As such they endeavour to answer questions about the key elements of learning. Theories of learning are numerous and different, and, to date, no single theory of learning has provided all the answers to all the questions raised. An understanding of some of the main theories of learning is useful because it provides us with an opportunity to examine or re-examine our own beliefs and assumptions about people, knowledge, motivation, environment, assessment and many other factors associated with learning.

The wide range of theories reveals much of what their proponents believe about the human species. The broad summaries contained in this chapter suggest that humans are variously seen as either extensions of other animal species or as a separate and distinct species with intellectual characteristics all of its own.

Classical behaviourism draws much of its theoretical base from experimental work on animals and extrapolates these findings to the learning process of humans. At the other end of the spectrum, represented here by Knowles, Brookfield and Schön, the adult human is capable of reflective, critical thought, different not only from other animals but also from younger members of the same species.

Learning theories teach us much about their proponents' views of people and the way they learn. The disciplines associated with critical thinking need to be used, in turn, to examine the cohesiveness and internal consistency of the theories themselves.

Numerous educational theorists and practitioners have proposed criteria by which learning theories should be interrogated. The fundamental questions that learning theories need to answer (adapted from Child 1986) are:

— How are the limits and scope of learning influenced by external factors, such as physical and social environment, and internal factors, including age, inheritance and disability?
— How does learning that takes place in early life influence learning in later life?
— Is there a relationship between the ways in which animals and humans learn?
— What is the relationship between physiological and psychological processes in learning?
— What is it that constrains or advances the achievement of practical or intellectual skills?
— How is learning influenced by motivational (internal or external) factors, including punishment?
— How can learning from specific activities and circumstances be generalised to others?
— What importance does 'understanding' have in the process of learning?

The learning theories summarised in this chapter represent broad schools of thought. In reality many educational practitioners adopt an eclectic approach, drawing on different theories to inform learning strategies that by necessity vary, depending on the nature of the subject, students, resources and other crucial factors.

## Behaviourism

Under this heading learning is concerned with individuals' response or 'behaviour' to a given stimulus. At the reflex level the reaction is an automatic response to the sensory stimulus, and at a slightly higher level the same response can be evoked through the association of a secondary or conditioned stimulus with the unconditioned stimulus: all nurses will have heard of Pavlov's experiments with salivating dogs. This type of learning is fundamental to habit formation, where some signal or stimulus sets off a series of activities, each reaction acting as a stimulus and creating yet another reaction. It may be fashionable to claim that such learning has no place in contemporary nursing education, and it is argued that today's student nurses learn best through enquiry, problem-solving, conceptualising theoretical situations and working out practical applications. For much nursing work this is appropriate, but there is also a need for an 'immediate motor response to a sensory stimulus'. Picture the nurse in a sudden, totally unexpected life-threatening situation. Her patient suddenly collapses and there are no vital signs; what nursing behaviours are now required? Does the nurse conceptualise the situation; is there time to consider and analyse the problem? These questions are rhetorical but they serve to remind teachers that undoubtedly the stimulus–response approach to learning has its place.

## Neobehaviourism

Behaviour modification, operant conditioning and positive reinforcement are all terms associated with this approach to learning, the main proponents of which include Skinner and Gagne. Learning, according to Gagne (1983), consists of sequential stages or a hierarchy of phases founded upon prerequisite abilities or intellectual skills. Many neobehaviouristic principles are appropriate to nursing education in the practice setting. Ward learning objectives and ward teaching programmes based upon the student's stage in training and level of attainment in previous practical placements are relevant factors compatible with Gagne's view of learning. Additionally Gagne very much stressed the importance of providing the student with immediate knowledge of his or her performance. Constant communication with the student, planning of feedback and regular evaluation of learning are therefore characteristic features of neobehaviourism. The ward sister or practical supervisor is effecting these principles of learning by carrying out pre-experience discussions with the student, identifying strengths and weaknesses, anxieties and expectations. Similar discussions or reviews may take place continuously during the student's placement and certainly at the end of the experience, where not only is an assessment of progress and attainment completed but also an evaluation of the experience is provided for the student.

## Gestalt theory of learning

Although very much an oversimplification of what is a complex process, the Gestalt approach may be summed up by the phrase 'learning through insight'. More accurately 'insight' is a fundamental component of the Gestalt learning process rather than a synonym for it — learning is the result of the student organising clues or components of a problem so that patterns emerge and solutions occur. This approach to education is very much concerned with problem-solving and discovery-learning methods. To the advocate of Gestaltism, the process by which a problem is solved and the learning that takes place during that process is often considered to be as important as the solution or outcome. It sometimes comes as a surprise to the inexperienced student nurse that the signs and symptoms of a particular disease or condition as described in a textbook are very rarely presented in such a way by the real-life patient. The student quickly learns, however, to observe, analyse and put together the clues that form the parts of the whole. With practice (and Gestaltists recognise that practice is important) the student begins to recognise patterns, appreciate relationships and perceive how problems can be solved and new conclusions reached. Thus learning is based upon awareness and understanding rather than on repetitive or habitual actions. Just as the signs and symptoms of an illness are different in real life from the textbook description, so too is the nature and course of the illness when witnessed in different patients. The student should now be able to discriminate between the behaviours of individuals and recognise the key features of an illness even though these may be masked and distorted by the patient's attempts to compensate or counteract the effects of illness.

## Cognitive theory of learning

This theory of learning is an extension of the Gestalt approach and seeks to build upon the insights of the student by stimulating the development of perception, understanding of principles and attainment of competences. The term 'cognition' relates to knowledge or knowing as opposed to feelings or activities, although it might be argued that in reality it is difficult if not impossible to isolate these three aspects or domains of behaviour. Compared with the stimulus–response focus of behaviourist learning, the student of cognitive theory will be attempting to interpret and develop some perception of the stimulus. This may necessitate referral to previous experiences, particularly those that might have had stimuli similar to those of the current learning situation. Bruner (1964), in supporting this approach, describes the spiral curriculum, which, although moving onwards, also circles back to previous experiences and understandings, building upon them and enhancing the appropriate issues, principles and values. Nurses may recognise the significance of the concept of the spiral curriculum in relation to the nine competences described by Rule 18(1) of the Nurses, Midwives and Health Visitors Rules Approval Order (DHSS 1983). All courses leading to initial registration must be designed to fulfil the appropriate learning objectives, learning opportunities and learning activities that will enable the student nurse to achieve and practise the aforesaid competences.

## Learning through reflection and student involvement

A number of educational theorists and practitioners have developed theories of learning that centre around the student's ability to develop critical thinking skills, which will, in turn, provide the mechanism for modifying performance in the light of experience. Whilst all different these theories each emphasise the central role of the student in the process of learning and the relationship between the student, the subject of learning and the person who enables or empowers the student to learn. Three influential writers in this area are Knowles, Schön and Brookfield.

Knowles 're-discovered' and actively promoted the concept of androgogy. This model assumes that the teaching offered to people in their late teens and beyond must be different from that offered to younger people if it is to be effective. In summary these differences are:

—    The adult student increasingly moves towards being self-directed rather than teacher-directed.
—    The adult's perception of experience is that it is part of them, unlike a child for whom experience is external to self.
—    Relevance of subject area is of far more importance to the adult learner than it is to the child.

Needless to say many of these assumptions have been vigorously challenged. This model has however been very influential in recent years (Squire 1987).

Schön's (1990) model of reflective practice points to the limitations of current rationality-based models of learning. He points to the need for people in practice to be able to respond to the majority of life situations that do not lend themselves to a predictable, rational approach:

'In the varied topography of professional practice, there is a high, hard ground overlooking a swamp. On the high ground, manageable problems lend themselves to solution through the application of research-based theory and technique. In the swampy lowland, messy, confusing problems defy technical solution. The irony of this situation is that the problems of high ground tend to be relatively unimportant to individuals or society at large, however great their technical interest may be, while in the swamp lie the problems of greatest human concern. The practitioner must choose. Shall he remain on the high ground where he can solve relatively unimportant problems according to prevailing standards of rigor, or shall he descend to the swamp of important problems and non rigorous inquiry?'

For Schön there is a critical relationship between the 'coach' and the student. He asserts that, in the realm of professional artistry:

'the student cannot be taught what he needs to know, but he can be coached'.

The emphasis is on students being able to see the consequences of their actions for themselves and determine the relationship between input and output. The role of the coach is as a 'guide' to the student as 'explorer' in this process.

Brookfield (1987) offers a discussion on the concept of analytical criticality and its place in adult life:

'Unless we become critical thinkers during periods of crisis, we are condemned to view our lives as constantly changing, essentially irrational sequences of random happenings that are out of our control. We are like psychologically shipwrecked voyagers, desperately clinging to whatever piece of psychic flotsam we can find as we are tossed in the turbulent seas of personal and social change.'

The teacher can model critical thinking in lectures, seminars, tutorials and practice situations to encourage students to adopt a similar frame of mind. Effective modellers have displayed most or all of the characteristics of:

— clarity;
— consistency;
— openness;
— specificity;
— accessibility.

These characteristics will be discussed further in the next chapter.

The above ideas about learning are important in discussions on nursing education for a number of reasons:

— They are congruent with a view of learning as a lifelong process and not just contained within the confines of a particular course or programme of study.
— They promote the idea of increasing self-reliance in the learner and decreasing dependence on the teacher. The nurse is therefore better equipped to participate in personal performance review and peer review in audit situations.
— With the development of community care and the changing skill mix on many wards, the qualified nurse is more likely to be working in isolation from other qualified colleagues. The need for professional self-reliance in isolated situations becomes greater as a result.

This introduction to some learning theories has sought merely to classify the different concepts and provide a framework within which the detailed factors relating to learning can be presented and discussed.

Educational courses in nursing, midwifery and health visiting may arguably be described as vocational, in that the student is in some cases additionally an employee contributing to the provision of a health care service or is in the process of specific preparation for employment. This chapter opened by stating that much learning would take place in the practice setting away from the theoretical confines of the classroom. The facilitation of learning in the practice setting raises particular challenges for student and teacher alike.

## Learning in the practical setting

Nursing education has a long history of providing practical experience for its students that has not always been directly related to theoretical instruction or motivated by educational factors. In recent years the statutory bodies have required the presence of concurrent theory and practice as a fundamental prerequisite to course approval. Pre-registration education programmes are increasingly becoming skills-based, with associated supportive theory. This has required educational planners to examine alternative models for curriculum building. When courses were heavily knowledge-based and theory preceded practical experience, a curriculum based upon a taxonomy as described by Bloom (1964) was ideal. The student followed a given theoretical concept through a series of levels, commencing with a basic knowledge and progressing through increasingly complex intellectual stages until the highest level of understanding was reached — all this in the absence of any realistic meaningful experience.

An experience-based course does not deny intellectual skills: indeed, the reverse is the case as it seeks to integrate them with both attitudinal and psychomotor skills to produce a student who can recognise the relationship between thinking, feeling and doing. When a student learns from a particular experience on a hospital ward or in a health care department, she does not just learn a piece of knowledge or physical skill or undergo a feeling in isolation each from the other. Any experience in which the student participates has a degree of knowing, feeling and doing. These three areas of behaviour are commonly referred to as domains — hence cognitive domain for knowing and understanding, affective domain for feelings and attitudes and psychomotor domain for physical actions or doing.

To try to devise a nursing course using these separate domains of behaviour, so that for each subject of the syllabus the knowledge part is taught first, then the practical aspects and finally the attitudes or feelings about it, may risk being seen as artificial and totally inappropriate for a course that has a strong vocational nature. Steinaker & Bell (1979) describe an approach to teaching and learning that claims not to break down human behaviour artificially into knowing, feeling and doing but to see human experience as a whole, bigger than the sum total of its parts. This closely resembles the Gestalt approach to learning and is compatible with Marson's (1979) plea to nurse educators and curriculum planners, reminding them that human behaviour is a holistic process and that all three domains of behaviour need to be integrated in a compatible and complementary manner for relevant learning to occur.

Where the main approach to learning consists of deliberate exposure of the student to situations or experiences, it is becoming increasingly referred to as 'experiential learning'. If an entire curriculum is based upon a sequence or series of levels of experience for which there are appropriate learning objectives, learning principles and learning strategies, it is understandable that Steinaker & Bell have called their approach to teaching and learning an 'experiential taxonomy'. There are five levels of experience in the sequence, commencing with exposure to the situation. Following exposure, which has to be seen as the fundamental basis to learning, there are four other levels, namely participation, identification, internalisation and dissemination. These are now briefly examined.

## Exposure to an experience

This first level of learning occurs when the student meets or is introduced to a specific situation. In the health care situation this may involve contact with a patient, visitors, staff members or a piece of equipment or machinery. At the exposure stage the student is using the senses to gain an appreciation and perception of the experience. Two options face the student; either to reject the experience, which will be difficult if it is a planned part of learning, or to accept further exposure and subsequent interaction. A positive response by the student leads to readiness for participation.

### Participation in an experience

This requires the student to become involved physically, emotionally and intellectually. A common practice in nurse education is for the student to rehearse the participation in an artificial or imitation setting, such as a skills laboratory, prior to carrying out the activity with a patient. This is thought to help in building the confidence of the student, although some teachers may suggest that it is only delaying the inevitable active involvement through which real learning takes place.

### Identification with the experience

Successful participation tends to produce emotional satisfaction and with it the desire to repeat the experience. This emotional satisfaction soon gives way to intellectual commitment and the student readily expresses opinions about the experience and is willing to share it with others, i.e. by talking about it to colleagues.

### Internalisation of the experience

When a new experience is accepted and practised at an intellectual level, it begins to be part of the lifestyle of the student, influencing both actions and attitudes. This may be something as simple as wearing a nurse's uniform and assuming some of the behaviours, values and beliefs associated with professional nursing. The effects may be only transitory to begin with, but as reinforcement occurs the experience becomes intrinsic to the behaviour of the student.

### Dissemination of the experience

The desire of the student to talk about and share her new piece of learning with others is already evident. At this final level of learning the student is now seeking to stimulate and inform others to become involved in the experience — she is beginning to teach.

## Some associated learning principles

So far reference has been made in this chapter to the main theories of learning, and the levels or stages through which a student may learn in a practice setting have been briefly described. If learning is to be more than an accidental outcome that is the result of good intention, opportunities for learning have to be planned, engineered and resourced. These issues will be addressed in more detail when the principles of teaching are considered in the next chapter, but if learning is to be meaningful and effective, a number of factors have to be present at the time of the learning experience. Some of these factors are internal or intrinsic to the student, e.g. feelings that are present, whilst other factors are external or extrinsic to the student, e.g. the influence of the environment. Rather than describe these factors or associated learning principles at random, a better appreciation may be achieved if they are examined as they occur at the different levels of the experience. For example exposure to an experience was described above as the first level of the learning process. What associated learning principles may be considered as important features at this early stage of the learning process? Certainly motivation is a key factor, and this incorporates, for instance, the individual's needs and drives, the desire to achieve, fear of failure and how others perceive one.

## Motivation, focusing, level of anxiety

Much has been written on the topic of motivation, and the needs satisfaction theory described by Maslow (1970) is probably the one with which most nurses will be familiar (Fig. 3.1). This theory suggests that as lower-level needs are fulfilled, there will be a drive to satisfy higher-level needs. Fig. 3.1 indicates that whilst nurses involved in learning have needs similar to those of other people, there are some specific illustrations, examples only, of the professional context with relation to Maslow's hierarchy. At the exposure stage of experiential learning, motivation is almost entirely of the extrinsic form and is concerned with creating a drive or a desire within the student to want to learn. For a student nurse this extrinsic motivation may be provided by enabling observation of a nursing skill being carried out in the practical setting rather than having it described in theory in a classroom.

Focusing is just an extension of motivation — it gives meaning to the stimuli that act as motivators. Using the above example of motivation, the nursing supervisor would direct the student's attention to the significant points to note whilst observing the nursing skill being carried out.

'Level of anxiety' refers to the student's state of emotional arousal. Most new situations have the potential for generating anxiety, the body's normal response, which is manifest through increased respiration, circulation and muscle tone. Such a degree of anxiety is a positive feature of learning, conducive to quick thinking and mental response. An excess amount of anxiety is of course detrimental to learning. If the student nurse in our example of observing a particular nursing skill has been told that she will be required to describe her observations to the rest of the student group, the anxiety then produced may be so great as to distract her observation and thinking. This will add further to her anxiety and may result in a completely negative learning situation. As the student progresses from the exposure level of learning and begins to participate actively in an experience, additional learning principles are required. Initial guidance, providing meaning and opportunity to explore, and creating chances for success are all important enabling features of the student's participation in the learning experience.

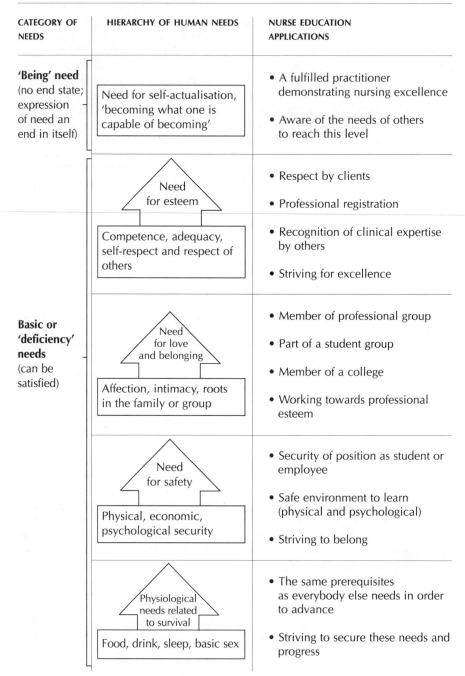

| CATEGORY OF NEEDS | HIERARCHY OF HUMAN NEEDS | NURSE EDUCATION APPLICATIONS |
|---|---|---|
| **'Being' need** (no end state; expression of need an end in itself) | Need for self-actualisation, 'becoming what one is capable of becoming' | • A fulfilled practitioner demonstrating nursing excellence<br><br>• Aware of the needs of others to reach this level |
| **Basic or 'deficiency' needs** (can be satisfied) | Need for esteem<br><br>Competence, adequacy, self-respect and respect of others | • Respect by clients<br><br>• Professional registration<br><br>• Recognition of clinical expertise by others<br><br>• Striving for excellence |
| | Need for love and belonging<br><br>Affection, intimacy, roots in the family or group | • Member of professional group<br><br>• Part of a student group<br><br>• Member of a college<br><br>• Working towards professional esteem |
| | Need for safety<br><br>Physical, economic, psychological security | • Security of position as student or employee<br><br>• Safe environment to learn (physical and psychological)<br><br>• Striving to belong |
| | Physiological needs related to survival<br><br>Food, drink, sleep, basic sex | • The same prerequisites as everybody else needs in order to advance<br><br>• Striving to secure these needs and progress |

**Fig 3.1**    Hierarchy of human needs (adapted from Roth 1990)

## Initial guidance, meaning, chance for success

Guidance during participation refers to the student having access to good briefing, supportive feedback, examples and illustrations, where appropriate, and a clear perception of the end product of the learning experience. Within the patient care environment the student may be preparing to participate in a patient assessment for the first time. The qualified nurse supervisor will have fully briefed the student and provided an opportunity for familiarisation with the relevant documentation. Preparatory activities may have included some rehearsal at asking questions and making accurate observations. At the same time as the student receives initial guidance, it is appropriate that a degree of meaning and understanding should be acquired. If the student can have a clear appreciation of the learning experience, its significance and importance, participation will then be enhanced and the degree of retention of knowledge increased. Because there is an understanding by the student of the reasons for assessing the patient's needs and how the information obtained will be used, the whole activity should then be that much more effective.

Both guidance and meaning are important contributors to ensuring that the student has the chance to experience success in the new learning situation. Where the chance to succeed in a learning activity does not exist or is very slim, participation in the experience will be non-productive. This will also be the case if there is the chance to succeed but the student has difficulty in recognising it. When success has been achieved, the student will not only seek to repeat the activity that brought about the success but will also aspire to further learning experiences of a similar nature. In the practical learning environment this may consist of the student repeating the activity with a different subject, i.e. carrying out a needs assessment on a different patient or reassessing the same patient at a subsequent date, this time with less guidance or supervision.

The emotional warmth and feeling of self-satisfaction that accompany success are highly significant factors in the movement of the student from the level of participation in a learning experience to the level at which identification with the experience begins to take place. It is through having specific feelings about an experience in the first place that the student can begin to examine it at an intellectual level. The learning principles that Steinaker & Bell (1979) associate with student identification with a learning experience are the personal interaction of that student, the knowledge of results and constant reinforcement.

## Personal interaction, knowledge of results, reinforcement

The successful participation in a new experience involves the development of an understanding and creates positive feelings, and examination of that experience at an intellectual level is made possible. Personal involvement with an experience is characterised by the desire to discuss it with others and further increase understanding, so having successfully carried out the patient care assessment, the student will wish to talk about the experience to other nurses.

A rapport will have been created between the student and the patient, and the desire to spend more time with the patient will be evident, the latter resulting from the student's feelings of now being personally involved with the patient and the need to acquire a deeper understanding about him.

Knowledge of results provides the student with insights into achievement, or lack of it, whichever the case may be. When the student can see the completed patient care assessment being used by the members of the nursing team as a basis for care planning, this represents a positive outcome. The student has evidence that learning has been successful and is acknowledged as such not only by peers but also by superiors.

Reinforcement is essential at this level of learning to ensure that practices resulting in positive and successful outcomes become a permanent feature of the student's professional behaviour. Skills transference is beginning to take place at this stage, and a good reinforcement strategy for the student nurse who is learning to assess patients' needs is to ensure that 'practice' is gained with patients who have different dependencies and needs. This will help to develop the newly acquired skills and create further opportunity for success. Reinforcement as a learning principle facilitates the transition from the level of identification with the experience to that of its internalisation; repeated practice in a wide variety of settings has ensured that what was an intellectual commitment to the activity is now becoming an automatic part of nursing behaviour.

### Overlearning, transfer (intrinsic), differentiation

The internalisation of a learning experience occurs with the incorporation of the experience into the student's life style, with the potential to influence feelings, attitudes and beliefs. This may be witnessed in its more overt presentation in, for example, the area of health education. The student nurse, having been exposed to the concept of the nurse as a health educator, has begun to participate actively in behaviours such as healthy eating, regular exercise, stopping smoking and mental relaxation. Having found this new life style beneficial, the student becomes committed to its principles and advocates them to others. As a role model for healthy living, the student is providing evidence of the internalisation of specific learning experiences.

What then is meant by overlearning? It sounds a somewhat derogatory term but it is in fact a very important principle of most learning processes. Overlearning is a type of reinforcement that gives the student the confidence and authority that comes with knowing or doing something very well. With overlearning the student is completely familiar with the skill or piece of knowledge and can use it readily. Now part of the work behaviour, it will be retained for future use and in addition become the foundation for transference to other activities. The student who has developed the skill of assessing patients' needs will be able to use the principles of assessment for problem-solving in a wide range of different circumstances.

Transfer of learning may best be described as a higher activity of the internalisation process and be typified by the student's ability to build upon established knowledge and skills for the development of new skills, and to formulate further concepts. This broadens the student's repertoire of experience and enables the conscious awareness of utilising or testing acquired knowledge in new situations. Having analysed the ability to assess patients' needs and plan appropriate care, the student may wish to see whether the same skills are applicable to other aspects of life: will the same professional skills apply in personal and social circumstances? All pre-registration nursing courses require the student to follow a planned sequence of different practical placements designed to provide a well-balanced appreciation of the caring specialisms and varied client groups. This programme of experiences also facilitates the learning principles of differentiation. After a period of caring for adult patients undergoing surgical treatment, the student may be placed in a day care centre that provides a facility for people with mental health problems. Can the student make adjustments to recently acquired knowledge and skills to meet the demands of this new learning environment? If the ability to analyse, assess and plan has been successfully internalised the student will quickly adapt to the new situation.

Returning to the student nurse who has adjusted her life style to reflect the total concept of healthy living, at the highest level of learning not only does the experience influence the behaviour of the individual but also she actively seeks to convince others of its merits and worth. This level of learning is referred to as *dissemination*, and its associated learning principles are *transfer* (extrinsic), *reward* and *motivation* (internal).

At this highest level of learning, the student now demonstrates high levels of competency. It is natural that a feeling of wanting to influence others now exists: the student has become the teacher and is shaping the behaviour of others — junior students, patients, relatives and other health care workers. Transfer of learning in its extrinsic form is the visible end product of the whole learning experience.

The student's reward is the satisfaction of disseminating knowledge and skills and influencing the values and beliefs of others. Assisting the junior student to participate in the assessment of and care planning for a patient carries with it the feeling of achievement and gratification, even though it is still a learning experience for the senior student.

The first learning principle referred to in this section was that of extrinsic or external motivation — that which would stimulate the student to want to learn. It is necessary to return to motivation to complete the account of learning principles, but now the source of the drive is intrinsic, within the student, rather than an external force. The need to provide further chances for success, reinforcing, rewarding and providing knowledge of results, still exists, but by now the student has experienced satisfaction and inner reward. The drive and desire to continue learning is now within the student, and provided that opportunities are created for continuing education and professional development, the motivation should be readily sustained.

The learning principle referred to are tabulated for easy reference, together with the corresponding level of learning, in Table 3.1.

Table 3.1 Learning principles (Steinaker & Bell 1979)

| Taxonomic level | Teaching role | Learning principle |
| --- | --- | --- |
| 1 Exposure | Motivator | Extrinsic motivation<br>Focusing<br>Anxiety level |
| 2 Participation | Catalyst | Initial guidance<br>Meaning — exploration<br>Chance for success |
| 3 Identification | Moderator | Personal interaction<br>Knowledge of results<br>Reinforcement |
| 4 Internalisation | Sustainer | Overlearning<br>Transfer (intrinsic)<br>Differentiated input |
| 5 Dissemination | Critic | Transfer (extrinsic)<br>Reward<br>Intrinsic motivation |

## Cooperative or competitive learning

When examining some of the important principles of learning, the use of terms such as motivation, chance for success, knowledge of results and reward is inevitable; they are proven key learning factors. Many cultures in the past have instilled in their young children a spirit of competitiveness whilst at the same time attempting to impress upon the child the importance of friendship, compassion and love for one's fellow person. Learning in some form or other appears to flourish in both sets of circumstances according to the particular individual. By that it is implied that some individuals learn some things best when there is a competitive nature to the learning situation. Other students seem to enjoy the group learning approach in which cooperation and interdependence are strong features. Which of these two attitudes to learning is best suited to the student in the practical setting? Care of patients and clients is claimed to be most effective when practised through a team approach — nurses, doctors, therapists and support staff working together to achieve a common goal. Each contributes specific skills, complementing the others. Can there be a role for the opportunist, competitor, aggressor or individualist other than that of an investor of these qualities into the team effort?

It will be argued in a later chapter that nursing education today should assume a more process-oriented approach whereby learning associated with human activities is a strong feature, enabling the student to grow. Constant feedback and reinforcement facilitate progress, with the knowledge that objectives and competences are being achieved. Nurse teachers spend much time and energy with new intakes of student nurses helping to create group cohesion, communication and fellowship. Interpersonal skills and social interaction are given a high profile not only to enable students to relate to patients and relatives but also, equally, to prompt cooperative learning and mutual support. Grading student performance leads to competitiveness, which Bevis (1978) suggests is antagonistic to the process approach to learning. This is also claimed by Biehler (1971), who in addition believes that it would be unlikely for one student to help another through a particularly difficult learning activity or event. Such attitudes are reinforcers of both high and low performance. If all students are provided with learning opportunities in which the probability of success is high, self-esteem is not threatened and team approaches are adopted, the competitive nature of the student may become modified and learning through cooperation may feature more strongly.

## Learning and memory

Principles of learning cannot be discussed without sooner or later making reference to memory and its associated components: remembering and forgetting.

We depend on memory in everyday life for our very survival. Without the use of memory, every encounter with particular stimuli or circumstances would require the learning of novel responses. In a nursing context this would mean for example that regardless of how many times a nurse had been involved in a cardiac arrest situation, each repeated episode would require the nurse to learn, as new, the resuscitation methods, emergency telephone numbers, location of emergency equipment and so on. This would clearly make life extraordinarily difficult and dangerous. The central theme of this section establishes a vital link between memory and learning. Rather than learning from scratch on each occasion, it is proposed that remembered experiences are built on and developed. In this way memory itself becomes a dynamic concept, with the student actively engaged in the process involved:

'You have to begin to lose your memory, if only in bits and pieces, to realise that memory is what makes our lives. Life without memory is no life at all . . . Our memory is our coherence, our reason, our feeling, even our action. Without it, we are nothing.' (Buñuel in Sacks 1985)

In addition to the example cited above, we are dependent on memory for our own self-image and self-concept. We are our memories in some respects. Our memories represent an active, living profile of our lives, skills, knowledge, relationships, prejudices and beliefs. Loss of memory, for whatever reason, casts us adrift from our past and present, as can be seen when a client sustains some traumatic or other damage to the brain.

It has already been proposed that memory is an extremely complex concept with competing and conflicting theories. Rather than examine these in depth, it is probably more helpful to consider a number of stages or processes involved in memory (Roth 1990):

— *Process of acquisition.* This process deals with incoming information. In addition to receiving information through the various senses, this information needs to be coded in such a way as to be stored in memory.
— *Process of retention.* This process is used to maintain information that has already been stored.
— *Process of retrieval.* This includes *recognition*, perhaps of a smell, a face, a taste or some other previous experience to a current experience, and *recall*, which is used to draw on stored information, perhaps in an examination or interview.

The language used to describe these processes strongly suggests that there is much that the student can do to develop memory and also much that the teacher can do to help the student. The ability to acquire, retain and retrieve information is crucial for students and clinical staff alike; the ability to forget is equally important. Techniques learned incorrectly are modified, in part, by unlearning or discarding information that is no longer helpful. For some this is as difficult as acquiring new information, for example when we can remember an old, replaced telephone number but cannot recall the new one.

For the student and teacher alike, there are some useful characteristics of memory that should influence approaches to learning.

— Single pieces of information are very rarely acquired in isolation from other events. A piece of information is acquired in context, and the context may considerably aid recall and recognition, so a principle that is presented by way of an anecdote or as part of a logical, reasoned presentation may be remembered more easily.
— New information is perceived through information already stored in memory. The actions of a student, teacher or member of staff will be interpreted against information already stored on that individual. A student who is frequently late on duty because of a hectic social life may, on the one day that he or she arrives late for quite legitimate reasons, find it quite difficult to convince the supervisor that this is not simply a continuation of previous behaviour. On the other hand the student may cause the supervisor to modify information already stored as a result of new information.
— Memory is influenced by many factors including attention, context, interpretation, motives and environment.

Whilst not denying that facts, information and experiences are forgotten over a period of time, there are obviously identifiable factors that can cause the forgetting process to slow down or, alternatively, accelerate. Similarly it is possible to develop mechanisms by which remembering can be enhanced and facilitated. Practice and revision readily spring to mind as agents of increasing remembering, particularly if carried out in a systematic manner. Buzan (1973) refers to the rehearsal of study notes after the first day, then after one week, one month and so on. This principle of helping memory is similar to that of producing immunity to disease through vaccination and booster injections, i.e. repeated doses/study at measured intervals increase immunity/retention.

This approach looks very attractive and no doubt can be effective, but how practical is it? Can a student so plan a learning strategy that it will enable the rehearsal of every new piece of information or allow timed repetition of experiences?

Ward managers and other health care practitioners will need to consider the significance of these factors relating to memory, remembering and forgetting when they are involved in the supervision of students in the practical setting. How do such factors apply in this type of learning environment, and what steps can the supervisor take to assist the student to retain and recall experiences and in addition relate them to concurrent theory?

Although learning is much more than committing to memory a series of related facts or practical activities, there are times when a sound memory and speedy recall of vital information are more valuable than the highly analytical problem-solving approach. The difficulty for the student nurse is often the infrequency with which new facts or skill items are encountered. Frequency and recency are important factors in the memory process, but quite often it may be things witnessed only once that are equally easy to recall. Very few students participate more than once during their training in the procedure for the removal of a specimen of cerebrospinal fluid from a patient. Why is it that years afterwards the student recalls exactly between which lumbar vertebrae the needle was inserted and can describe the appearance, pressure and specific gravity of normal cerebrospinal fluid and perhaps even remember Queckensted's test? There are, indeed, a number of reasons, which are applicable to most situations in which accurate retention may be desirable.

Firstly, there is the 'sense of occasion' if it is the first time that the experience is to be entered into, which is almost always an emotional as well as cognitive learning experience. Because of these factors the student can often re-live the experience in the imagination. This second feature of memory retention, i.e. imagery, can be very intense, particularly if the emotional component of the learning happened to be particularly strong, either in a positive or negative way. It is a commonly held belief that circumstances involving negative emotions such as fear or anger are readily forgotten or not retained well in the memory, i.e. they are suppressed. Many qualified nurses can give very clear examples of experiences memorised for life as a result of a less-than-happy emotional situation as a student. Whilst not doubting the truth of this, one would not advocate the generation of negative emotions within the student as a means of facilitating memory retention.

Finally, in the discussion of learning principles, it is appropriate to consider what responsibilities, if any, students have towards their own learning and their development of study skills. Now, more than at any other time in recent years, the teacher or course designer is challenged to meet the needs of students with vastly differing experiences of life, education and preferred styles of learning. The demographic profile among pre-registration student groups continues to show an increase in the number of mature students. For some students their course represents their first reintroduction to *formal* learning for many years. Others will have recently graduated from university or undertaken vocational education programmes for careers other than nursing. It is worth noting, however, that the preferred learning styles of students are often assumed rather than established in any teacher–student dialogue. What it is reasonable to expect is that the student will recognise and practise new techniques of learning and begin to assume increased responsibility for self-directed study. In this respect the role of the teacher, which will be further discussed in Chapter 4, becomes as much associated with helping the student to develop the skills associated with learning as with imparting knowledge and demonstrating skills. It is important that the student is able to develop the sophisticated skills of appropriate discrimination, for example between right and wrong in infinitely varying circumstances, between transience and permanence in respect of nursing knowledge and practice and between high and low priorities.

Whilst learning is an innate part of the human entity, the contribution that the teacher is able to make to the process is akin to what Schön refers to as coaching, enhancing the performance of students through enabling them to learn effectively and efficiently through experience. These issues will be further described in Chapter 4.

## References

Bevis O M (1978) *Curriculum Building in Nursing.* St. Louis: Mosby

Biehler R F (1971) *Psychology Applied to Teaching.* New York: Houghton, Mifflin Company

Bloom B S (1964) *A Handbook of Educational Objectives, the Cognitive Domain.* New York: McKay

Brookfield S (1987), *Developing Critical Thinkers; Challenging Adults to Explore Alternative Ways of Thinking and Acting.* Milton Keynes: Open University Press

Bruner J S (1964) *Toward a Theory of Instruction.* Massachusetts: Belknap Press

Buzan T (1973) *Use your Head.* London: BBC Publications

Child D (1986) *Psychology and the Teacher.* London: Cassell

Curzon L B (1990) *Teaching in Further Education.* London: Cassell Education Limited

DHSS (1983) *Nurses, Midwives and Health Visitors Rules Approval Order 1983* (Cmnd 873). London: HMSO

Gagne R (1983) *The Conditions of Learning.* New York: Holt, Rinehart and Winston

Krathwohl D *et al* (1968) *A Handbook of Educational Objectives. The Affective Domain.* New York: McKay

Marson S (1979) Objectives, markers along the way. *Nursing Mirror,* 8th August

Maslow A H (1970) *Motivation and Personality.* New York: Harper and Row

Roth I (1990) *Introduction to Psychology.* Hove/Milton Keynes: Lawrence Erlbaum/Open University

Sacks O (1985) *The Man Who Mistook His Wife for a Hat.* London: Picador

Schön D (1990) *Educating The Reflective Practitioner.* San Francisco: Jossey Bass

Simpson E (1966) *The Classification of Educational Objectives. Psychomotor Domain.* Illinois: University of Illinois Press

Squire G (1987) *The Curriculum Beyond School.* Sevenoaks: Hodder and Stoughton

Steinaker N W & Bell M R (1979) *The Experiential Taxonomy.* New York: Academic Press

UKCC (1986) *Project 2000, A New Preparation for Practice.* London: UKCC

# 4
# The Principles of Teaching

**Defining teaching**

The difficulties experienced in trying to define teaching mirror, perhaps not surprisingly, the difficulties experienced in trying to define learning. Theories of teaching and the roles of teachers reveal their proponents' beliefs about the nature of human beings in the same way as theories of learning do. Definitions of teaching range from the mechanistic (Curzon 1990):

'a system of activities intended to induce learning, comprising the deliberate and methodical creation and control of these conditions in which learning does occur'

to 'reflection in action' (Schön 1987):

'coach and student convey messages to each other not only, or even primarily, in words but also in the medium of performance. The student tries to do what she seeks to learn and thereby reveals what she understands or misunderstands. The coach responds with advice, criticism, explanations, descriptions — but also with further performance of his own.'

As with theories of learning, one is unlikely to encounter a definition of teaching that satisfies all teaching circumstances with all students. Each of the definitions cited above has its strengths and limitations. Because of the prescribed nature of practice, learning outcomes and the need to 'organise' learning opportunities in the context of a busy and complex workload, the practice-based teacher will find much to commend Curzon's definition. Its limitations are, by the same token, highlighted by the complexity of learning the 'craft' of professional nursing and the varying learning styles and needs of individual students, which are more obviously acknowledged in Schön's model of 'reflection in action'.

The value of teaching, in the sense that it means imparting knowledge and skills or instructing, is itself disputed:

'Teaching, in my estimation, is a vastly over-rated function.'

'Teaching and the imparting of knowledge makes sense in an unchanging environment. This is why it has been an unquestioned function for centuries. But if there is one truth about modern man it is that he lives in an environment that is continually changing. The one thing I can be sure of is that the physics that is taught to the modern day student will be outdated in a decade . . . We are, in my view, faced with an entirely new situation in education where the goal of education, if we are to survive, is the facilitation of change and learning.' (Rogers 1983)

This discussion surely highlights the enormous tension experienced by all 'teachers' involved in the education of nurses. On one hand the teacher must work with prescribed learning outcomes produced by the accrediting body. In turn, these outcomes may be underpinned by statute. On the other hand the teacher must creatively account for the almost unimaginable complexity of the environment, the student and teacher workload, not to mention an ever changing world of health care practice.

These complexities are enhanced for the practice-based teacher when asked to ensure that what is learned by the student is at a particular level of study. It is difficult enough for full-time educational staff to determine what consolidates, for example, 'diploma' level teaching or assessment in a classroom. How much more difficult it is to clearly understand and recognise the characteristics of diploma level practice.

Whatever the complexities are surrounding teaching in the practice setting, there is widespread agreement that appropriately supported practice placement experience is an essential part of the education of nurses. The debate over the relative merits of theoretical and practical education in nursing programmes has been brought into sharp focus during the implementation of the Project 2000 proposals. Research conducted on behalf of the Department of Health identified the complexities of this new approach to nursing education for practice-based teachers of students.

Whilst offering a generally optimistic view of Project 2000 developments, this research (Jowett et al 1994) identified the following problematic issues:

— concerns expressed by nurse teachers about their practice-based role;
— differentiation between the 'rostered' and 'supernumerary' status of students;
— the quality of links between education and service;
— time available to practice-based nurses for teaching student nurses;
— the emphasis placed on innovations in pre-registration programmes with limited preparation for existing practitioners;
— the increasing complexity of practice-based assessment;
— supervising and assessing students who would achieve a higher level qualification than they themselves hold.

The teaching role of the practice-based nurse has become more complicated at a time when the nursing role generally has also become more complex. The demands of service and education are increasing as the rate of change in both areas is becoming more rapid. In the next few sections of this chapter, some of the main elements of the teaching role of the clinical nurse will be discussed.

## The teacher's role in clinical practice

Qualified nurses in clinical practice are reticent about adopting the title of teacher, yet when asked to describe their job, the terms 'supervising students' or 'having students on the ward' would feature strongly. Halsbury (1974) recommended that ward sisters' salaries should reflect their roles as teachers and assessors of student nurses. This initiative was further developed in 1988 when the Department of Health announced its clinical grading structure for nursing and midwifery staff (Table 4.1), in which the descriptions of each of the clinical scales set out their clinical, education and management characteristics. In so doing the Department of Health in some respects established a hierarchy of teaching and supervision roles in clinical practice. Recent research (Jowett *et al* 1994) would suggest that there is still some way to go:

'It seems increasingly unrealistic to regard student supervision and assessment as an activity to be "tagged on" to the existing full-time workload of already over-stretched practitioners.'

Even within these guidelines the potential education or training roles and activities that an experienced nurse could be involved with are many and varied:

— member of curriculum development team;
— mentoring junior qualified colleagues;
— member of examination board;
— auditing clinical practice;
— ward-based assessor/examiner;
— production of ward learning objectives;
— preparation of student progress reports;
— completion of course evaluation reports;
— implementing ward teaching programmes;
— teaching and assessing role development.

As the delineation between 'theory' time and 'practice' time has become clearer (all pre- and many post-registration courses now set out the hours of each), so the purpose of this time needs to be more clearly focused. In the past practice-based teachers have sought to set up pseudo-classrooms in the clinical setting to provide what, with the best of intentions, has been described as 'proper teaching' for students. The result of this is to extend the theoretical input to students at the expense of the sole legitimate purpose of nursing education, which is to enhance the practice of nursing. The challenge to practice-based teachers is to enthral the student with the quality of practice demonstrated by skilled practitioners who have themselves reached the level

Table 4.1    Clinical grading structure (derived from Department of Health 1988)

| Scale | Professional development requirements | Teaching and supervision characteristics |
|---|---|---|
| Scale C | Normally holds second level registration | (i) Expected to demonstrate own skills to new or junior staff |
| Scale D | Holds first level registration or second level with specialist experience, qualification or supervising responsibilities | (i) Demonstrates procedures and supervises qualified and unqualified staff |
| Scale E | Holds first level qualification and a further registerable qualification or skill acquired through experience | (i) Expected to supervise junior staff and teach qualified and unqualified staff including pre- and post-registration students |
| Scale F | First level qualification and experience at E or conditions as for E grade | (i) Standard-setting; supervision and deployment of staff<br>(ii) Teaching nursing and non-nursing staff |
| Scale G | Minimum level for district nurses, CPNs, community mental handicap nurses, health visitors and community midwives, or continuing responsibility for ward, etc. | (i) Standard-setting<br>(ii) Manages a ward or caseload<br>(iii) Supervision, deployment and teaching of staff and/or students |
| Scale H | Statutory supervisor of midwives<br>OR<br>Holds a recordable teaching qualification<br>OR<br>Qualified practical work teacher/ fieldwork teacher | Manages more than one ward or caseload |
| Scale I | Required to hold a recordable teaching qualification<br>OR<br>Clinical specialist with extensive knowledge<br>OR<br>Is managerially responsible for more than one ward or its equivalent in the community | (i)   Provides advice within and outside profession<br>(ii)  Supervises, deploys and develops staff<br>(iii) Designated statutory supervisor of midwives<br>(iv) Assessing training needs<br>(v)  Planning, implementing and evaluating the education and training of pre- and post-registration students in classroom and/or practice setting<br>(vi) Provides clinical advice and support to other staff |

of dissemination. The student who is undertaking a clinical placement where the emphasis is placed on excellence in nursing, regard for patients and respect for their dignity is more likely to be excited by the prospect of participating in such activity. The characteristics associated with excellence in nursing as experienced by patients are, perhaps unsurprisingly, the same characteristics that student nurses report on positively when reflecting on placement experience.

Discussions on who is the most appropriate person to work with students in the practice setting still abound. The grading criteria in Table 4.1 above suggest that practising nurses have a key role to play in this process. Other bodies such as the ENB have expressed the need for nurse teachers to retain a clinical orientation. They have perhaps recognised the need for nurse teachers to play an active part in the supervision and education of students in the practice setting. The point is raised here because as changing skills mix formulae are developed in practice settings and the diversity of practice settings is continued, nurse teachers may increasingly be the only constant link between theory and practice for the student. This book is however orientated towards the educational development of practice-based nurses whose teaching role is described in the clinical grading structure, all staff from grade C upwards having a clear teaching and supervisory role as an explicit part of their nursing role.

In the recent past the emphasis has been placed on practice-based nurses gaining, through a variety of educational programmes, the skills necessary to teach and assess student nurses in the practice setting. ENB Courses 998 and 997 have particularly emphasised this need, and the demand for such programmes continues to be high.

There have been numerous and varied approaches to preparing nurses to fulfil their role in nurse education. These have ranged from three-day art of examining courses to more sophisticated attempts to provide the ward sister with some teaching skills. Many managers have acknowledged the worth of courses such as the City of Guilds Further Education Teacher's Certificate, and have assisted staff to attend local colleges on a day-release basis. The ENB Course 998/997 was the first nationally validated course expressly designed to meet this specific need. Finally, when making the strong claim that the practising nurse is the most appropriate and credible person to fulfil the clinical teaching role, it must be added that employers have of course to find the resources to fund this activity. It may well be that in future only those employers who are willing and able to prepare their 'practical teachers' adequately will receive the statutory approval to run nurse education courses.

Subsequent chapters of this book deal very specifically with the teaching methodology, describing such terms as role model, mentor and facilitator. Here will be discussed the very simple conceptual model of nursing described by Chater (1979), showing three interlocking circles that represent the patient or client, the nurse and the environment or setting in which care is given (Fig. 4.1). Adding a fourth interlocking circle representing the student would seem to provide a very apt conceptual model of practical nurse teaching (Fig 4.2).

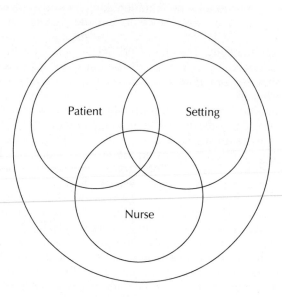

Fig 4.1    A conceptual model of nursing (Chater 1979)

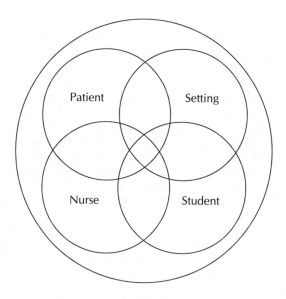

Fig 4.2    A conceptual model of practical nurse teaching

This conceptual model clearly suggests that nurse, patient and student have a relationship that is interactional and therefore interpersonal, each party having roles and responsibilities as well as needs and expectations. The balance and emphasis of these aspects differ of course between the participants, but each has something to give and receive from the others.

The concept of an experiential curriculum has already been advanced when learning principles were described. Applying the same five stages of the experiential taxonomy to teaching roles and strategies as were applied to learning principles makes it possible to match appropriate teaching approaches with student learning needs. This seems particularly relevant in the practical teaching and learning setting where students are participating in realistic experiences.

### The nurse supervisor as motivator

The first level of the experiential learning process is characterised by the student being exposed to the subject of the learning situation. Accompanying this level of learning are the principles of external motivation, focusing and management of anxiety. The corresponding teaching role is that of motivator. For a student nurse in the initial stages of the course it is essential that supervision by the qualified nurse should provide not only opportunities to learn but also safe ones — total protection so that anxiety levels are not such that they interfere with learning in a negative way.

Perhaps for the teacher in the clinical setting being a motivator for the student at the exposure level of learning is not very much of a problem. Clearly the student nurse is already highly motivated: having competed for a place on the course, she is only too eager to commence learning in the reality of the patient environment. However three years plus is a long time in the life of a young adult, and initial enthusiasm tends to wane sooner or later. It is at these times that the skill of remotivating becomes invaluable. Being able to create within the student the desire and need to progress from one level of learning to another is not always easy. An early positive, secure rapport between the student and supervisor is necessary, without the need for threats or excessive demands. Well-directed observations, together with realistic demonstration and problem identification, may help to stimulate the student. Knowing that a student has particular strengths can be useful to the supervising nurse when planning learning opportunities. It is vital that the exposure level of learning is managed well in terms of student motivation, as unless there is a desire to begin to participate in the learning experience, the student will make no progress.

### The nurse supervisor as catalyst

The word 'catalyst' is the only meaningful word to describe the role of the nurse at this next level of student learning. The purpose or aim is to assist the process of change along the learning continuum, i.e. from observation of an experience or activity to participation in it. In chemical terms a catalyst is a change facilitator that speeds up a reaction between two or more substances. Using this analogy the teacher, together with appropriate resources, enables a change to take place between the student and the object of the learning experience. This provides the student with an opportunity to develop not only an intellectual commitment or understanding but also an emotional attachment.

During this transitional period the practical teacher must maintain a good level of motivation in the student and protect her from the risk of failure. Close supervision, prompting where necessary and at all times keeping the student well informed about the 'what', 'why' and 'how' of the nursing activity are characteristics of an effective role model. If the teacher fails to act as a catalyst at this participation level of the learning process, many things could happen, which may not only slow learning down but even prevent it from taking place. A student who is told to obtain a specimen of urine from a patient and is shown how to test the specific gravity but not given any explanation of why it has to be done does not have the total picture; a part of the experience is missing and with it the potential for developing that growing commitment upon which the next stage of the learning process depends. Equally bad is the situation in which a student is given a full explanation of why a nursing activity is carried out but is inadequately prepared for or supervised in its execution. This situation is potentially dangerous. A bad experience for the student at this stage can bring a complete halt to the learning process.

As with the previous level of learning where the teacher took on the role of motivator, the catalyst function is of an extrinsic nature. The student has a somewhat passive role still and is even being manipulated in many of the learning situations. Through repeated participation in well-planned activities, however, the student will become both intellectually and emotionally attached to the experience, and at this stage the teacher's role will need to change again.

## The nurse supervisor as moderator

In simple terms a moderator is someone who sees that things are kept within certain limits, preventing extremes from occurring or being brought to bear on a situation. The student is now at the stage of learning of which 'ownership' of the skills, activity or experience is claimed. Identification of the learning experience has taken place and the student is incorporating the new learning into professional behaviour. During this identification level the student will seek to test newly acquired skills: will they 'work' in differing circumstances with different patients? It is at times like this when the student, not yet experienced, wants to experiment that the supervisor has to ensure 'moderation' in practice. The student at this stage begins to demonstrate the principles of reflective practice (Dewey 1974):

'[the student] has to see on his own behalf and in his own way the relationship between means and methods employed and results achieved. Nobody else can see for him, and he can't see just by being "told", although the right kind of telling may guide his seeing and thus help him see what he needs to see.'

Although the nurse supervisor is now playing a more passive role, it is essential that the learning opportunities should be available and provide a meaningful sequence of experiences for the student. Positive reinforcement must be given, and the role model is consistently questioning and suggesting appropriate student actions, clarifying any problem areas as they occur.

Some qualified nurse supervisors may find this particular role difficult to come to terms with. They are being urged to *teach* student nurses, yet at significant stages in the learning process, a passive role is recommended. This is understandable because of the traditional concepts of the teaching role, but at this level the teacher is manipulating the student through a learning experience and controlling the learning environment.

For the supervisor there is the tension between the learning needs of the student and the safety needs of the patient. The supervisor has a primary allegiance to patients, ensuring that no harm occurs to them as a result of the students' learning-in-action. At the same time the student needs to be able to take risks and experiment in order to learn and develop. The supervisor therefore needs to assess the need for risk-taking and the possible consequences of such risks, minimising the possibility of harm to both patient and student.

Sensitive handling of the student is called for, assisting with such interactive needs as she may have in terms of sharing the positive experiences and receiving appropriate feedback. These new behaviours, which the student demonstrates and develops a commitment for, are now becoming assimilated into the growing repertoire of acquired skills. The teacher will assist by helping with the selection of relevant information and its use, giving the student regular indications of progress and achievement.

### The nurse supervisor as sustainer

The level of learning for which the particular teaching role is best suited is that of internalisation. Having identified with a particular skill or nursing activity and 'tested' it in a variety of situations, it can now be reproduced without any conscious effort. The skill has become a learned behaviour for the student, a permanent feature of the range of necessary competences that will lead to qualification. As with the previous level of learning, the teaching role is relatively passive, although much support is still necessary as the student requires constant approval, particularly where recently acquired skills are being used in new situations. It is important that the student should recognise the appropriateness of the action and see it as a positive contribution to the care of the patient/client.

A word of caution is necessary at this point. Where very specific behavioural objectives have been prepared for students, there could be some variation in initial performance, the degree of motivation, the student's own interpretation and the different response levels that will influence the learning outcomes. Provided these responses are within acceptable parameters, the nurse supervisor can engineer necessary adjustments. An important feature of the sustainer role is the requirement to provide the student with additional scope for practice, extending her experience and enabling the transference of skills. Perhaps rather than manipulating the student, the nurse supervisor is adjusting the learning environment, creating different learning opportunities. New experiences can seriously challenge the student, stretching her ability to adapt and adjust. As a sustainer of learning, the teacher will be re-motivating whenever necessary, promoting creativity and encouraging innovation, yet remaining sensitive to all the demands being made upon the student.

The risk assessment role referred to above continues to be a feature of the supervisor's behaviour. In seeking out new learning opportunities for the student and encouraging innovative practice, the supervisor (UKCC 1992):

'must, in serving the interests of patients and clients and the wider interest of society, avoid any inappropriate delegation to others which compromises these interests.'

### The nurse supervisor as critic

At the beginning of this account of the different roles of the nurse supervisor in relation to the student's level of learning, it was evident that the teacher adopted an active stance, which gradually became more passive as the student progressed along the learning continuum. Such a shift in emphasis within the teacher–student relationship is common, particularly in further and higher education. The statutory bodies for nursing have in recent years advocated a curriculum strategy whereby initial teacher-directed approaches gradually give way to student-centred learning and eventually to self-directed study. This model would appear to be completely appropriate to adult learning until the question of the student moving on to a new learning experience occurs. Because self-directed learning is the mode at this stage, are new learning activities left to chance or should the teacher again assume an active role? In the model being offered here, the highest level of learning, described as dissemination, is accompanied by a teaching role that places the nurse supervisor firmly back into an active position relative to the student. The nurse supervisor is now a critic, appraising, evaluating and advising the student. With objective criticism and by asking questions or posing further problems, the teacher prepares the way for new learning experiences.

### The nurse supervisor as role model/mentor

The previous chapter referred to the characteristics of effective role modellers. The role model/mentor is effective when displaying the following behaviours (Brookfield 1987):

— *Clarity*. The student is able to identify, without doubt, what it is that makes a role model effective.
— *Consistency*. Modellers do not vary their responses to the student on the basis of unjustifiable and irrational stimuli. The modeller is just and fair, a stable reference point in a changing environment.

— *Openness.* The mentor demonstrates honesty and integrity, being open about her knowledge and skills and the limitations of both, sharing uncertainty and being self-critical and open to external criticism.
— *Specificity.* The mentor behaves in such a way as to allow for 'interpretive imitation'.
— *Accessibility.* The modeller is not only physically accessible, important though that is, but also encourages enquiry by not being intimidating.
— *Communicativeness.* Mentors can clearly articulate their actions through a full repertoire of examples, metaphors and analogies.

This model is more cyclical, in that the highest level of learning is often the precursor of new experiences, the motivation to learn this time perhaps being intrinsic rather than an extrinsic provision via the teacher.

This sequence of teacher roles in relation to the levels of learning within an experience is of course a model or framework for the teacher, and it is readily acknowledged that roles may need to change or undergo modification within the prevailing circumstances. A simple representation of this model is shown in Fig. 4.3.

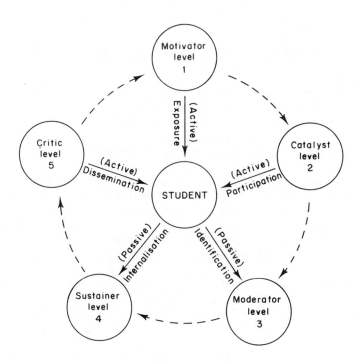

Fig 4.3     Teaching roles in relation to levels of learning

## The nurse supervisor as coach

This aspect of the nurse supervisor's role is not particularly associated with any one part of the experiential taxonomy, but the characteristics of coaching change with the emerging confidence of students as they develop. Schön (1987) describes the extent to which:

> 'groups of students . . . are often as important to one another as the coach. Sometimes they play the coach's role and it is through the medium of the group that the student can immerse himself in the world of the practicum . . . learning new habits of thought and action.'

## The curriculum process in the practical setting

Until recently all pre-registration nursing courses had been founded upon a syllabus published by a statutory body. Project 2000 (UKCC 1986) notes amongst recent major changes in nurse education the shift away from prescribing the exact knowledge to be obtained. This move is concerned with developing the responsibility of curriculum process to the individual schools and giving support and advice through the use of guidelines and general principles. The syllabus for courses leading to registration in Part 1 of the Professional Register (general nursing) was formally withdrawn by the ENB in 1986 (Circular 1986/65/ERDB). It was replaced by guidelines published in the previous year (Circular 1985/19/ERDB) to assist schools of nursing in the design and development of curricula to meet the requirements of Rule 18(1) of the Nurses, Midwives and Health Visitors Rules Approval Order 1983 (DHSS 1983); this rule is reproduced in Fig. 4.4. The licence and flexibility permitted by the statutory bodies for selecting teaching and learning strategies by which the 'product' can be achieved is welcome; it can however make demands upon curriculum designers and the students' supervisors.

The need to ensure a curriculum that reflects contemporary care practices and values means that course planning teams should have adequate clinical representation. In order to ensure a complete understanding of the courses being developed, clinical staff should be encouraged to contribute to all aspects of the course and not just the unit or that part of the programme in which they are personally involved. The progression of the student nurse from day one of the course is planned in a sequential manner, and different learning and teaching principles are required that are dependent upon the stage of the student's development within the course. Not all competences will be attained at the same rate: some e.g. health promotion, will be achieved relatively early in the course, whilst those relating to teaching and management will be acquired nearer its end. Because of the very real potential for causing the nurse supervisor confusion and misunderstanding, it is vital that the curriculum design team should, in consultation with nurse supervisors, devise appropriate teaching strategies for each unit of practical experience and the theory concurrent with that experience. This will usually take the form of written objectives designed to enable the student to achieve a goal or aim for that part of the course. When put into the form of questions to be answered, the nurse supervisor needs to know the following:

— What purpose or purposes should be achieved by the student in the particular practical placement?
— What experiences can be provided to enable the purposes to be achieved?
— How can these experiences be effectively prepared and arranged?
— How can the attainment of these purposes be measured?

These questions are still as relevant today as they were almost 40 years ago when referred to in Tyler's (1949) work on curriculum development. Child (1986) comments on Tyler's use of the word 'experience' instead of 'content', reflecting that the term 'experience' concerns not only the subject material taught but also the process by which the learning takes place. Child summarises the four questions posed by Tyler as objective, content, method and evaluation.

---

18(1) Courses leading to a qualification the successful completion of which shall enable an application to be made for admission to Part 1 of the register shall provide opportunities to enable the student to accept responsibility for her personal professional development and to acquire the competencies required to:

(a)   advise on the promotion of health and the prevention of illness;

(b)   recognise situations that may be detrimental to the health and well-being of the individual;

(c)   carry out those activities involved when conducting the comprehensive assessment of a person's nursing requirements;

(d)   recognise the significance of the observations made and use these to develop an initial nursing assessment;

(e)   devise a plan of nursing care based on the assessment with the co-operation of the patient, to the extent that this is possible, taking into account the medical prescription;

(f)   implement the planned programme of nursing care and where appropriate teach and co-ordinate other members of the caring team who may be responsible for implementing specific aspects of the nursing care;

(g)   review the effectiveness of the nursing care provided, and where appropriate initiate any action that may be required;

(h)   work in a team with other nurses, and with medical and paramedical staff and social workers;

(i)   undertake the management of the care of a group of patients over a period of time and organise the appropriate support services;

related to the care of the particular type of patient with whom she is likely to come in contact when registered in that Part of the register for which the student intends to quality.

---

Fig. 4.4 UKCC training rules (Nurses, Midwives and Health Visitors Rules Approval Order, DHSS 1983)

## Objectives

At the practical experience level an objective can be defined as a statement describing what the student nurse will be able to do after completing the practical placement; it is a comparison of the behaviour of the student after the learning experience with that before it. Because of this reference to behaviour, these objectives are more commonly referred to as behavioural objectives.

When describing objectives Curzon (1990) differentiates between the general objective and the specific objective. The general objective is sometimes referred to as the terminal objective because it states the behaviour expected at the end of a unit of learning or a practical placement. Similarly specific objectives may be described as development objectives because they are achieved during the course unit and their sum total results in the achievement of the terminal objective. Some advocates of behavioural objects will be even more specific in describing the expected behaviour. In addition to a description of the observable behaviour, the teacher may state the conditions under which the behaviour is to be achieved and furthermore the precise criteria for successful attainment. Translated into nursing practice a behavioural objective concerning the administration of drugs may look like this:

On completion of this learning exercise the student will be able to:
(a) carry out a ward medicine round
(b) under the supervision of a qualified nurse
(c) and in accordance with the authority's policy.

Just as there are advocates of this approach to learning and the rigid setting of objectives, there are those who severely criticise behaviourism in any shape or form. They argue that to specify predetermined outcomes to all learning situations is more akin to training, whereas education, whilst not denying the end product, is just as much concerned with the process by which that product is achieved. What nurses have to decide is whether nursing is a profession or a vocation. If it is the latter, training with behavioural objective is perhaps an appropriate learning approach. In the practical nursing setting the wide diversity of learning opportunities, combined with the complexity of individual differences in patients or clients, would seem to render the construction of strict behavioural objectives expensive of time and effort. The number of behavioural statements that could be involved might be too numerous to cope with, and neither do behavioural objectives take into account the unique nature of the individual student and her previous experiences.

The experiential approach to curriculum design and process, whilst acknowledging the necessity of objectives, links them to the broader experience rather than to a narrow behavioural outcome. This allows for and indeed encourages the individuality of the student, recognising that learning speeds, motivation, special interests and expectations vary widely amongst course members even where there is a common goal or purpose.

Perhaps in such a diverse subject as nursing there is room for both behavioural and experiential objectives. The emergency situation that threatens life requires the nurse to be very specific in her behaviour towards the patient, using a skill learned through very precise behavioural objectives. The building up of a supportive and therapeutic relationship with a newly bereaved relative can perhaps be very rarely achieved using behavioural learning objectives.

There is no denying that teaching and learning objectives of some form or other help to bring some structure to most types of educational course, providing a framework upon which teaching strategies and assessment criteria can be based. At the practical level in the clinical setting, the qualified nurse who fulfils the supervisory role in basic nurse education must play a prominent part in the formulation of objectives. These objectives must be realistic and meaningful and truly reflect the care practices taking place; it is futile for theoreticians to design ideal objectives that bear no relationship to the practical reality in which the student is required to gain experience.

It may be helpful at this stage to provide the reader with specific examples of different types of objective as they might appear in the curriculum structure of a basic nursing course (Fig. 4.5).

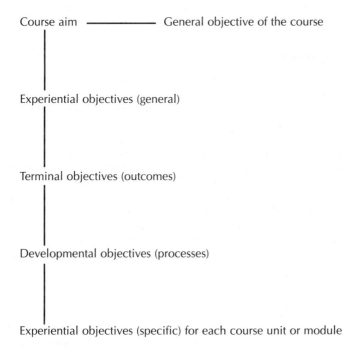

Fig 4.5 Curriculum model showing sequence of objectives

*The course aim*

To produce a contemporary nurse who can respond to consumer demands and needs using problem-solving techniques that reflect a wide range of technical, behavioural and intellectual skills.

*General objectives of the course*

The course will provide opportunities to enable the student to acquire the competences specified by Rule 18(1) of the Nurses, Midwives and Health Visitors Rules Approval Order 1983 (DHSS 1983; Fig. 4.4 above).

*Experiential objectives (general)*

The course will expose the student to nursing practices using appropriate role models who reflect nursing competency:

— The course will enable the student to participate in experiences with role models competent in the giving of total patient care.
— The course will encourage the student to identify with competent care giving, as practised by the role model.
— The course will enable the student to internalise the skills of a competent nurse.
— The course will prepare the student to disseminate the competences described in Rule 18(1) (Fig. 4.4 above).

*Terminal objectives (outcomes)*

— The student will be able to accept responsibility for personal professional development.
— The student will advise on the promotion of health and prevention of illness.
— The student will recognise the situations that are detrimental to health and well-being.
— The student will be able to assess a patient's nursing requirements.
— The student will devise nursing care plans, with the patient's cooperation where possible.
— The student will implement planned care and teach other care team members whilst coordinating their activities.
— The student will review and evaluate care given to patients.
— The student will work effectively in a multidisciplinary team setting.
— The student will manage the care of patients, organising appropriate support services.

*Development objectives (processes)*

— The student will demonstrate an understanding of situations detrimental to physical, emotional and social wellbeing and will show a responsibility towards the promotion of health.
— The student will demonstrate an ability to give total nursing care to a

specific patient whilst under the supervision of a qualified nurse.
— The student will develop this ability and be able to assume responsibility for the nursing care given.
— The student will become competent in implementing and evaluating nursing care for a group of patients.
— The student will develop the ability to manage the total care of a group of patients.
— The student will consistently demonstrate the nursing competences described by Rule 18(1) (Fig. 4.4 above).

## Experiential objectives (specific to a course unit)

When designing objectives for a particular part of a course, it would appear desirable to write these in terms of nursing behaviours, wherever possible associated with one or more of the nursing competences of Rule 18(1) (Fig. 4.4 above). The following are examples of such experiential objectives taken from an early course unit of a basic student general nursing course.

**Exposure level**   'The student has observed the qualified nurse's use of the skills of listening, responding and clinical observation which are needed to complete patient assessment.'
This first level of learning, i.e exposure to an experience, in this example is linked with the competencies (c) and (d) of Rule 18(1).

**Participation level**   'The student has participated in the planning of nursing care under the supervision of a qualified nurse.'
In this example the student has progressed to the second level of learning, i.e. participation, and competency (e) of Rule 18(1) is the focus of study.

**Identification level**   'The student demonstrates an awareness that many situations in health care provision may be detrimental to the individual's health.'
This objective, pitched at the third level of experiential learning, is concerned with competency (b) of Rule 18(1) and requires the student to have developed an understanding of health hazards, institutional problems and safety risks when caring for patients and their relatives.

**Internalisation level**   'The student can explain the purpose of care given and its relation to the level of dependency of the patient.'
The student who has 'internalised' a particular experience has incorporated the required skills into the nursing behaviour. In this example competency (f) of Rule 18(1) provides the basis for the learning objective.

**Dissemination level**   'The student can advise the patient and relative on matters of health promotion by acting as a role model.'
At this highest level of learning the student can be observed to be 'teaching' others about their experiences and demonstrating skill in their professional behaviour. The objective given here relates to competency (a) of Rule 18(1).

## Course content at the practical level

Having defined the teaching and learning objectives for the course as a whole and for each of its component parts, the next stage in the curriculum process centres on the selection or identification of appropriate experiences and subject content. For the nurse supervisor in the clinical setting, this will very much depend upon two things: firstly, the objectives that the student must achieve in relation to the stage of training, i.e. first year, second year, third year, and, secondly, the nature of discipline of the experience, i.e. medical, orthopaedic, psychiatric, and so on.

In a curriculum that is substantially skills-based, the knowledge or theory components are secondary to and supportive of those skills required to achieve the objectives of a course unit. The qualified nurse who is charged with the supervision of student nurses will need to give attention to questions such as:

— What is the student to learn?
— How is it to be learned?
— Why is it being learned?
— How much attention must be given to it?

These questions relating to curricular process are by no means complicated or profound, but until recently it is unlikely that many qualified nurse supervisors would have been required to provide answers to them. Perhaps a cardinal rule for all teachers at the practical level is to present material or information to a student only in such a way that it has to be used or acted upon immediately (Bevis 1978).

What the qualified nurse supervisor must resist at all costs is the temptation to teach 'pet' subjects to the student. There is no point in a student nurse being able to recite the names and functions of the 12 pairs of cranial nerves whilst gaining practical experience in the community with patients requiring mental health care.

Concurrent theory and practice is advocated by the statutory body, and this should be interpreted as the provision of background information and knowledge to support the practical experiences as they occur or are managed. The situation in which a student is denied the experience of accompanying a patient who is to undergo a liver biopsy because the anatomy and physiology of the liver has not been taught in the school should not occur. As a student receives new experiences in the clinical setting, she should be prompted and guided to acquire the relevant support material and information so that a total meaning is obtained for that experience and it can form a link in the educational chain. Accepting that some of the experiences and the associated knowledge will be specialised, the nurse supervisor should nevertheless give significant emphasis to the course topics. These may differ slightly depending upon the course but ought to revolve around such themes as health concepts, care models, the nursing process and personal service.

## Teaching strategies (method)

Learning principles were considered in the previous chapter and teacher roles were looked at in the earlier part of this one. Probably the most important feature of the curriculum process is teaching strategies, as these represent the interface between students and curriculum philosophy and cannot be discussed in isolation. It is the amalgam of learning principles, teacher roles and teaching strategies that sets the scene for the teacher–student relationship and with it the whole teaching–learning process. All too often a curriculum is prepared with detailed attention to learning objectives and subject content and is then handed over to the teacher without any attempt being made to suggest appropriate teaching strategies. Whilst this is unfortunate if it happens to the professional teacher, it must be considered inexcusable and totally unacceptable for the nurse supervisor to be placed in such isolation.

Fortunately when using an experiential approach to teaching and learning, this should rarely happen. The teaching strategies considered appropriate at each level of learning are proposed in association with the learning principles, and simultaneously the role of the teacher in the teacher–learning activity is suggested. Nevertheless, as Kelly (1982) warns, it is the teacher, in this case the nurse supervisor, who has the task of bridging the final gap that might exist between theory and practice. Ideally all teachers and supervisors who are to participate in curriculum implementation should have been involved in its design. This can be partially achieved when designing nursing courses by involving clinically-based nurses who are to be the supervisors of students in the appropriate stage of course design. Two purposes can be achieved in doing this: firstly, by contributing directly to course design, the nurse identifies with the course and becomes involved with its ownership, and, secondly, the role-specific needs of nurse supervisors can usually be revealed at this juncture and the necessary development training and role preparation planned.

The description of teaching strategies may be better understood if they are considered in the context of nursing themes, i.e. care models, nursing process and health concept. It will also be necessary for the reader to recall the table of learning principles in the Chapter 3. Just as certain principles are found to be appropriate to particular learning levels, so too are specific teaching strategies. Such strategies are now described using the levels of learning as the sequence for presentation. The activities of living model described by Roper *et al* (1983) will be used as the example of a nursing approach, mainly because it appears to be the most common model used in the UK health service.

*Teaching strategies at exposure level*

**Goal setting**    The nurse supervisor will introduce the concept of daily activities of living to the student and endeavour to create an incentive within the student to explore the concept in detail.

**Data presentation**    Using the student's own experiences of daily living a profile or checklist of activities can be developed.

**Demonstration**    Some of the underlying principles of daily living activities can be demonstrated by the supervisor using examples of patients' behaviour, students' own behaviour or media resource material.

**Directed observation**    Selecting a number of activities of living, e.g. eating, breathing, personal cleanliness, etc., the student can analyse in detail how an activity is carried out.

**Data exploration**    The student should now follow up the analysis by interpreting findings and extracting relevant information for care planning purposes.

These five teaching strategies are designed to shape the students' observational skills and let students become more aware of their own experiences of living whilst examining the life processes of other people.

### Teaching strategies at participation level

**Recall**    As part of the preparation for participation, the student should review the information acquired at exposure level. Comparison of one's own needs for fulfilling activities of living and independence with those of patients will help in understanding the dependence–independence continuum.

**Expanding information**    The information gathered can now be expanded through discussion with the supervisor or peers in such a way that experiences are shared. Questions can be asked relating to the identification of resources needed to meet the dependency needs of patients, and plans for helping patients to fulfil their activities of living can be proposed, formulated and examined.

**Role-play**    Although this teaching strategy is usually more appropriate to the classroom, it may have occasional use in the practical experience setting. The supervisor may wish to rehearse with the student such activities as patient admission, interviews, counselling and other interactive processes. Role-play may prove to be the best preparatory method, provided that the rehearsal is not too artificial or unreal.

**Practice participation**    Supervised practice can now follow in the reality of the patient setting and basic nursing activities carried out working alongside an experienced role model. In addition to physical manipulation skills, the student must be encouraged to practise observational and communication skills.

**Ordering**    Following participation in assessing, planning and implementing basic care designed to assist patients with activities of living, the student should now analyse the particular role played. Additional information will have been collected in transit and mistakes will have been made. This information can now be arranged, sequenced and structured into a planned framework for future practice.

## Teaching strategies at identification level

**Active participation** The student should now be ready for more sustained practice whilst still under the supervision of a nurse. Although experience is now being gained with all components of the nursing process, emphasis for the student will still be around the application of caring skills.

**Using information** It should now become apparent to the student that existing information can no longer meet the diversity of the caring situations being experienced. Additional reading will be necessary, and the student will begin to use information and interpret it to meet new circumstances. Patients have different degrees of dependence and need: some are keen to participate in self-help whereas others enjoy being dependent. Increased skills of observation and communication will enable the student to use information more effectively. This principle is well supported by Taylor (1985) who suggests that the skills of information processing should be acquired at an early stage in training in order to facilitate the use of new content and assist the student in the analysis of new data.

**Interactive discussion** Opportunity must be provided by the supervisor during the allocation to practical experience for the student to discuss future expectations and anticipated progression. It is important for the student to be able to express ideas, discuss new information and review outcomes of practice. During ward meetings, discussion designed to clarify problem areas, identify difficulties and allow expression of opinions will help with the reinforcement of learning. Debate can be centred around some of the less physical aspects of living, e.g. expressing sexuality, assisting patients to communicate and caring for the dying. The student will need some feedback on the achievement of progress, and the supervisor can use this interactive discussion to advise the student of weaknesses and, equally important, reinforce strengths.

**Hypothesising** As the student's skills and confidence increase, so will the ability to ask questions in relation to the carrying out of care: 'When I discussed my particular interest in painting with Mrs. Green, she said it was also her main hobby and she has now expressed an interest to do some painting in the evenings when the ward is quiet; I wonder if I can discover Mrs. Brown's hobbies or interests and encourage her to participate in something creative or diversional.' The student is now beginning to examine in depth the activities of living and see connections between meeting these and the promotion of independence. Assumptions based upon reasoning are now being produced.

Before proceeding to the teaching strategies appropriate to the higher levels of learning, it is necessary to do a quick stock-take of the progress made along the teaching–learning continuum. The student has by now undergone a substantial period of practical experience, participating in the nursing care of patients whilst using a particular model of care. During this time the student will have gathered, analysed and acted upon a wide range of information. Ideas will have been generated and tested against reality under the supervision of a competent role model, and degrees of success will have been experienced. The student should now be able to demonstrate an understanding of the 'activities of living' approach to care and how it is implemented using the nursing process. It is important that the student not only understands the model of care but is also able to appreciate that many other models of nursing exist.

## Teaching strategies at internalisation level

**Skill reinforcement**    As the student progresses through the course, gaining experience with different patient or client groups in different clinical settings, existing skills will be tested in new settings and reinforcement of the more productive elements of care will take place.

**Creative expression**    Just as theoretical knowledge can be enhanced by providing an opportunity for practical application, so too can skills be strengthened, enriched and reinforced by encouraging the student to write about experiences and talk to others about them in a group or seminar. By doing this the student is giving expression to internalised learning and sharing both with peers and supervisors. Being able to talk about experiences adds a further dimension to the learning and is valuable preparation for transition to the dissemination level.

**Role-play and simulation**    The testing of skills amongst peers can be further extended by the use of role-play and simulation. Because the student is now both emotionally and intellectually committed to the concept of nursing models and health promotion, the use of advanced role-play can enable full expression and interpretation of these concepts. The student can gain practice in developing the role of health educator by trying out a range of health promotion strategies under the safety and security of her supervisor's protection. It is equally important for the student to appreciate and understand the consumer's feelings and point of view as a receiver of health education and nursing practices. With the use of simulation the student can stand in the patient role whilst a peer or supervisor plays the role of health promoter. Role-play is an effective expression of internalised learning, whilst simulation is an expression of understanding and therefore probably less threatening for the student. Internalised behaviour during simulation can be allowed expression without risk of ego damage.

**Comparative analysis**    Although the student has by now experienced a number of different patient settings in which to carry out nursing care, these experiences will probably have had a degree of similarity in that they may all have taken place within a particular type of hospital setting. Can the student utilise her nursing skills in a totally different environment with a very different patient/client group? How will the student adjust and modify her approach to an acutely mentally ill patient in a psychiatric unit or to a domineering ex-patient in his own home? Such situations will test the student's critical thinking and problem-solving abilities. The nurse may have achieved the skills of meeting the personal hygiene needs of a helpless patient confined to bed but will the same techniques succeed with a severely depressed suicidal patient? This difference in the type of experience enables the student to compare and contrast the utility of the nursing model and how the nursing role has to change in approach and application. The student will need to analyse critically the similarity and differences that a new client group or care environment creates and, with the help of a skilful role model, broaden her knowledge base and add to her repertoire of skills.

**Summarising**   The internalisation of the activities of a living model is almost complete. Because learning sequences have been well planned and learning has taken place by intent rather than by accident, the student can possibly review the process that has been undertaken. Any activity that helps the student to summarise or conclude the whole concept of activities of living will be most helpful in rounding off the internalisation end of learning. The presentation of a seminar paper to the ward team or the submission of a written assignment to the supervisor serves this purpose.

*Teaching strategies at dissemination level*

**Reporting**   Dissemination is totally a student-centred activity; it cannot be demanded by a supervisor, or rather, more accurately, it should not be demanded. The student, having internalised the competencies of carrying out total patient care is, in comparative terms, an 'authority' on the subject. The student should not only wish to share experiences with others but should also be positive in advocating them to nursing colleagues. Additionally the student at this level should be willing to defend her work and deal confidently with objective criticism.

**Oral presentation**   As the student's desire to advocate her learning to others grows, not only will opportunities be used as they arise but also the student will seek to create opportunities. Whilst carrying out nursing activities with patients, the student may offer health-promoting advice with regard to diet, exercise and smoking. Similarly with relatives the student may tactfully introduce health concepts into the general conversation. Although these two activities would appear to be very similar, there is a distinct difference in emphasis: with the patient the nurse will be seeking to change behaviour whereas with relatives the emphasis is usually more informal than prescriptive.

**Dramatisation, group discussion, seminar**   In addition to written reports and oral presentations, there are a number of dissemination strategies available to the student. Many situations of a social or psychological nature lend themselves to dramatisation, particularly in areas where a health education message is desired. Dramatisation differs from role-play in that the student creates a theme and writes the script, which is then acted before an audience. Although this has limited use as a teaching strategy in the clinical setting, the nurse supervisor may wish to use it in health education activities for patients and relatives.

The strategies of coaching and role modelling have been described earlier in this chapter. They have an important part to play throughout all levels of the experiential taxonomy.

Group discussion at ward meetings and seminars presentation to team members are social activities in which the student can participate. Through debate, an attempt can be made to influence others and also to test beliefs and values against the opinions of others. Seminars or group discussions may give rise to new ideas and extensions to concepts that have previously eluded the care team.

In concluding the description of teaching strategies, it must be emphasised that rarely do students complete the five levels of learning in one course unit. For some of the more complex concepts an entire course is needed to enable the student to progress from exposure to dissemination and competency. A summary of the teaching strategies relative to the levels and principles of learning is given in Table 4.2.

Table 4.2    Summary of learning and teaching strategies (after Steinaker & Bell 1979)

| Taxonomic level | Learning principles | Teaching strategies | Teacher role |
|---|---|---|---|
| 1 Exposure | Extrinsic motivation<br>Focusing<br>Anxiety level | Goal setting<br>    motivation<br>    presentation<br>Demonstration<br>Directed observation<br>Data exploration | Motivator<br>Information<br><br>Coach<br>Role model |
| 2 Participation | Initial guidance<br>Meaning — exploration<br>Chance for success | Recall<br>Expanding information<br>    base<br>Role-play<br>Practice participation<br>Ordering | Catalyst<br><br>Coach<br>Role model |
| 3 Identification | Personal interaction<br>Knowledge of results<br>Reinforcement | Active participation<br>Using information<br>Interactive discussion<br>Hypothesising<br>Testing | . Moderator<br><br>Coach<br>Role model |
| 4 Internalisation | Overlearning<br>Transfer (intrinsic)<br>Differentiated input | Skill reinforcement<br>Creative expression<br>Role-play — simulation<br>Comparative analysis<br>Summarisation | Sustainer<br><br>Coach<br>Role model |
| 5 Dissemination | Transfer (extrinsic)<br>Reward<br>Motivation (intrinsic) | Reporting<br>Oral presentation<br>Dramatisation<br>Group dynamics<br>Seminar | Critic<br><br>Coach<br>Role model |

## Assessment within the teaching strategies

Although specific chapters (5 and 6) are devoted to the subject of assessment, it is necessary here to say a few words about the practical nature and the assessment function in relation to the teacher strategies that have just been described.

### Assessment at the exposure level of learning

At this first level of learning the nurse supervisor provides learning experiences designed to stimulate the student's interest, with a view to monitoring her to seek further exposure to the experience and begin to interact with it. Assessment involves the student and judging her levels of interest and interaction. It may be possible even at this early stage to assess initial understanding and attitudes towards the experience. Informal methods such as ward team discussions, question and answer and nurse supervisor observations are appropriate during this learning stage.

### Assessment at the participation level of learning

Participation implies a conscious decision by the student to become involved in the learning experience. Again observation by the nurse supervisor is an obvious assessment method, provided it is acknowledged that at this stage much of the learning may not be overtly expressed. To reveal covert learning the supervisor would need constantly to question the student to determine levels of learning, and this is neither practical nor desirable. A better approach would be to vary the opportunities so that students can make choices and interact with a number of alternative solutions, thereby revealing more overtly a comprehension of their participation.

### Assessment at the identification of level learning

Identification with the learning experience is achieved when the student begins to convert the satisfaction of participatory achievement into intellectual commitment. At this level there is a tendency for overt expression of the learning, the student often wishing to share her learning with others. Assessment at this stage must be used to reinforce learning and reveal to the student some degree of achievement, and it must also identify attainment of goals in the form of unit objectives. Assignments, surveys and projects are most probably the methods of choice because their outcomes can be used in a formative way and they can additionally be criterion referenced.

### Assessment at the internalisation level of learning

With internalisation learning has been incorporated into the behaviour of the student, part of the life style influencing both actions and attitudes. Assessment at this level should attempt to reveal an ability to solve problems, analyse situations, interpret findings and express concepts. Surveys or small research studies, presentation of care studies and case histories are all activities that will enable the student to demonstrate such characteristics of learning and which can also measure the achievement of objectives.

### Assessment at the dissemination level of learning

Dissemination, the highest level of learning, involves the outward expression of learning. The student is now the 'teacher'; she has the desire to stimulate and inform others, even to impress her learning upon others. Because the bulk of this behaviour is overt, it is assessable. The supervisor will be looking for not only the ability to solve problems, analyse and interpret situations and data but also the degree of influence the student has on others. What are her values, and how well developed are her judgemental skills? Does she have the ability to act as advocate and counsellor? Assessment will involve submission of critical analyses of care plans and evaluations by the student to her supervisor. The student will readily demonstrate an ability to teach and behave as a role model to others. Student self-assessment, peer assessment and the desire to set objectives for continuing development all confirm that the dissemination level has been achieved.

## Conclusion

As the student progresses through the levels of learning from exposure to an experience to its ultimate dissemination, so the supervisor passes from being an observer, questioner and measurer to an appraiser of the student, with the task of judging to what extent the learning experiences in the clinical setting have influenced the student's behaviour. The impact of good, or bad, teaching lasts long beyond the duration of any single course of study. Exposure to good teachers will ensure that the student internalises good values and will ultimately influence the student's experience as the process of disemination unfolds. The student will be encouraged to continue a lifelong approach to learning with resultant benefits to the experiences of patients and students alike. Exposure to bad teaching may result in a rejection of the experiences and place a block on further exposure to similar experiences, or worse still the student may internalise the values of poor role models and disseminate these into the nursing profession.

## References

Bevis E O (1978) *Curriculum Building in Nursing.* St Louis: Mosby

Brookfield S (1987) *Developing Critical Thinkers: Challenging Adults to Explore Alternative Ways of Thinking and Acting.* Milton Keynes: Open University Press

Chater S (1979) In Bower F L & Bevis E O (eds) *Fundamentals of Nursing Practice: Concepts, Roles and Functions.* St. Louis: Mosby

Child D (1986) *Psychology and the Teacher.* London: Cassell

Curzon L B (1990) *Teaching in Further Education.* New York: Holt, Rinehart and Winston

DHSS (1983) *The Nurses, Midwives and Health Visitors Rules Approval Order 1983* (Cmnd 873). London: HMSO

DHSS (1988) *New Clinical Grading Structure for Nurses, Midwives and Health Visitors.* London: HMSO

Dewey J (1974) *John Dewey on Education: Selected Writings.* Chicago: Chicago University Press

Halsbury Lord (1974) *Report of the Committee of Enquiry into Pay and Related Conditions of Nurses and Midwives.* London: HMSO

Jowett S *et al* (1994) *Implementing Project 2000.* Slough: NFER

Kelly A V (1982) *The Curriculum, Theory and Practice.* London: Harper and Row

Rogers C (1983) *Freedom to Learn for the 80s.* Columbus: Merrill

Roper N *et al* (1983) *Using a Model for Nursing.* Edinburgh: Churchill Livingstone

Schön D (1987) *Educating the Reflective Practitioner.* San Francisco: Jossey Bass

Steinaker N W & Bell M R (1979) *The Experiential Taxonomy.* New York: Academic Press

Taylor S G (1985) In Riehl-Sisca J (ed.) *The Science and Art of Self-Care.* Norwalk, Connecticut: Appleton-Century-Crofts.

Tyler R W (1949) *Basic Principles of Curriculum and Instruction.* Chicago: University of Chicago Press

United Kingdom Central Council (1986) *Project 2000: A New Preparation for Practice.* London: UKCC

United Kingdom Central Council (1992) *The Scope of Professional Practice.* London: UKCC

# 5
# The Principles of Assessment

There is no more contentious subject in education than that of assessment. In 1984 Minton was right in asserting that 'Teachers and Society are content with relatively unsophisticated achievement tests which often do not differentiate between the many things they may be measuring together'. Since this time, however, the political spotlight has played on education in general and on the assessment of its effectiveness in particular. The aim, as with the whole quality imperative dealt with in Chapter 2, has been to increase Britain's share of wealth through the creation of a highly skilled and flexible workforce able to cope with the new technologies and quality-led approaches.

In the education and training arena the overall aim was the achievement of an increase in the standard of general education. In schools the National Curriculum introduced compulsory testing of children at the ages of seven, 11 and 14. More young people were to proceed to higher education in order to raise the percentage of British graduates in the workforce to that exhibited by countries with an unarguably successful economic record. The old 'binary divide' between universities (with their traditional academic bias) and polytechnics (which focused on imparting the knowledge and skills required by employers) has been removed, thus increasing the attractiveness of vocational degrees. Simultaneously both old and new universities were enjoined to ensure that their courses equipped people for the values and technology of the last years of the twentieth century. At the lower end of the ability scale there was a drive to ensure that a larger proportion of young people left school at least literate and able to benefit from the training opportunities that employers, with government incentives, were to offer.

With the publication of the Manpower Services Commission's review of educational qualifications in England and Wales (MSC 1986) and the subsequent White Paper *Working Together — Education and Training*, vocational training was grasped and brought under the umbrella of the National Council for Vocational Qualifications (NCVQ). Few at the time realised the impact that this paper would have on the future of education. The innovative feature of National Vocational Qualifications (NVQs) was that they were defined not by completion of a given length of study but by the demonstration of competence — a shift in emphasis from teaching to assessing. We will return to the subject of NVQs later in the chapter but will meanwhile consider other pressures for change in the field of assessment, which originated within the profession itself.

Firstly, with the introduction of Project 2000, it became a requirement that all pre-registration courses should be taught (and assessed) to higher education diploma level. Secondly, the ENB has since 1990 required that all courses be continuously assessed. Finally, the introduction of the ENB's Framework and Higher Award has created the possibilities of replacing 'courses' with more flexible 'pathways' through which individual students can steer a coherent course, resulting in their demonstrating the achievement of the 10 key characteristics (Fig. 6.3 below). Together these criteria have changed the face of nursing assessment and brought new challenges to those entrusted with the task of judgement.

## Defining assessment

Assessment suffers from being well known and, in some respects, little understood. This is reflected in the numerous and conflicting definitions of assessment and the number of terms that are used synonymously with it. Recently concepts of 'profiling' (Broadfoot 1986) have been added to those of examinations and tests. For some assessment is an omnibus term that includes all the processes and products that describe the nature and extent of learning, and additionally includes measures of the social and economic value of the curriculum. For the purposes of this discussion, assessment is defined as:

'Measurement that directly relates to the quality and quantity of learning and as such is concerned with student progress and attainment.'

This deliberately restrictive definition assumes assessment to be distinct from, but subordinate to, evaluation, which is concerned with measuring the overall worth of the curriculum and not exclusively student progress. The concept of evaluation is considered separately and in detail in Chapter 10.

## Why assess?

It might seem to be common sense that students undertaking a course of training should be assessed, but to assume unthinkingly that students should be examined denies a complex debate concerning the purpose of examinations and indeed the need for examinations at all. Satterly (1981) undertook a comprehensive study of the issues involved, and although the debate focuses in particular on primary and secondary education, the issues raised are of equal relevance to nurse education. Objections sometimes raised against examinations are outlined below.

*Assessment is a political activity that preserves the social order of society.*
It is alleged, particularly by those on the political left, that examinations limit

opportunities, thus perpetuating the existing hierarchical structure of society and resulting in the application of labels that determine the individual's opportunities in life. Despite the abolition of selection at the age of 11 and the creation of comprehensive education, the education system labels students as high, medium, low and non-achievers through the awarding of examination certificates. The possession of three A levels of a suitable grade permits entry to university, whilst non-possession of GCSE qualifications denies the opportunity to be a sales assistant in our most prestigious high street chain stores. Extremists claim that assessment is 'a tyrannical means of persuasion, coercion and social control' (Rowntree 1987). At the very least it is the means of one group of people (professionals) exercising control over others (students).

Whatever additional criteria are used to select student nurses, the statutory educational requirements defined in the Nurses, Midwives and Health Visitors Rules (DHSS 1983) are 5 GCSEs at grades A–C. There can be no doubt that 'good' intelligence is required for registration, and the stated number of qualifications requires intelligence. However such achievement also demands appropriate social circumstances such as a stable and supportive home environment and, increasingly an issue in the 1990s, a secondary school that is able to afford appropriate teaching and learning materials and opportunities. Again the many enrolled nurses who have successfully achieved registered status bear testimony to the fact that the required standard can be achieved by those leaving school without formal certificates. It is true that there exists a test to give entry opportunities to those who would otherwise be debarred, but it is expensive and time consuming to administer. To access this test in many areas, the ability to pay to sit the test becomes an additional assessment hurdle, and the frequency with which it is offered is in most cases driven by recruitment patterns rather than by high-minded notions of providing equal opportunities to those recognised as being disadvantaged within the educational system.

*Assessment favours the middle class, which is to the disadvantage of other groups and too often interpreted as differences in innate potential.*
Throughout education there is an awareness of middle class bias. Certainly it has been demonstrated that children from the lower social classes do less well than their middle class friends in examinations and tests. Factors influencing this are claimed to be the possession of a greater vocabulary, easier access to books and reading materials, the availability of private space in which to study at home, and the greater rapport between middle class parents and school teachers (also largely drawn from the middle classes). These factors are all equally pertinent in nursing education, which, with its entry requirement, already de-selects many of the socially deprived. A factor frequently overlooked in considering assessment is that the process of initial selection is the first assessment. Those involved in the interview process must be aware of the 'halo effect' by which means a well-spoken, middle class candidate may be assumed by an equally middle class interviewer to possess many other positive attributes such as, for example, high intelligence or greater sensitivity.

*Assessment is limited to relatively trivial educational objectives whilst the most important aims of schooling are inaccessible to testing.*
Whilst it is possible to take formal school qualifications in many more areas than formerly, there is no attempt to measure, for example, social interaction, for the award of a GCSE in conversation. The same accusation can be levelled against assessment in nursing. Sims (1976) showed that ward managers rated psychosocial incidents highly when rating effective performance, but procedural incidents predominated when describing ineffective behaviours. Lankshear (1990) demonstrated that whilst clinical assessors believed that among the most important qualities of a student nurse were interest in learning and in their patients, a caring disposition and the possession of good communication skills, the same assessors felt unable to fail students in the overall ward report unless the issue was concrete, definable and unequivocally related to patient safety.

*The results of assessment have an uncanny knack of being self-fulfilling.*
Two distinct types of expectation can be influenced by assessment: the teacher's expectations of students and the students' expectations of their own future performance. In the latter case the results of assessment are incorporated into individuals' concepts of themselves. Early in a course of training, depending on the results of assessments, students develop a success or failure identity. Consequently they may, with limited justification, believe themselves to be 'good' or 'bad' at a particular subject or skill. The student who succeeds expects future successes — for 'nothing breeds success like success' — and is motivated accordingly. In contrast the student who fails may withdraw from further attempts to learn.

   Those responsible for teaching and assessing develop expectations of the performance of their student nurses; these are based partly on explicit assessments and partly on implicit influences such as the student's appearance, social background and speech. These expectations are then reflected in the type of work allocated to the student, the difficulty of a question asked in the classroom or the level of concern and interest demonstrated in respect of an individual student. These expectations are, consciously or unconsciously, transmitted to the student who consequently performs in the way we expect him or her to perform. Of the 'self-fulfilling prophecy', Satterly (1981) observes:

   'The overall result of a teacher's assessment can be detrimental for those students who are set low expectations and correspondingly damaging for those who, because of an unrealistically optimistic assessment are set levels they are quite unable to fulfil.'

*Assessment encourages the student to develop the styles of thought and intellectual 'tricks' required by tests and therefore inhibits the development of other skills.*
Miller & Parlett (1974), following a study of students at the University of Edinburgh, suggest that students perceive examinations to be a game that is irrelevant to real life, and consequently they study the rules of the game in order

to be good at it. One group of students they called 'cue seekers'. These individuals scrutinise previous examination papers, discover their teachers' main interests and prejudices and actively attempt to engage teachers in conversation in the hope of detecting hints of likely examination questions. Subsequently they invest their energy in rehearsing probable examination questions. These 'cue seekers' contrasted with 'cue conscious' colleagues, who would pick up any hints dropped by teachers but did not make a career out of analysing previous papers and attempting to elicit teachers' stands on various topics. The last group, comprising approximately 50% of students, were oblivious to hints and unwilling to study 'form' and were consequently dubbed 'cue deaf'. Whilst cue seeking is quite legitimate, it can be argued that in thus concentrating their studies, students who so engage themselves are diluting their level of achievement. One may question whether the professions can tolerate practitioners with significant gaps in their knowledge base caused by a calculated guess that 'it won't come up'.

*Assessment inevitably takes place in a role-relationship. This is antithetical to a truly educational setting where encounters between teachers and students are interpersonal.*
An assessment is a judgement made by someone about someone else, which of necessity invokes a hierarchical and authoritarian relationship between assessor and assessed. Knowles (1973) describes this preoccupation with teacher-dominated assessment as 'progressively recessive', denying students responsibility for learning and inhibiting self-criticism, self-assessment, self-reliance, independence and creativity. The judgemental and authoritarian 'I–It' relationship between teacher and student was for many years a feature of pedagogy — the art and science of teaching children. In contrast androgogy — the art and science of teaching adults — demands an equal and non-judgemental relationship between teacher and student, a relationship of mutual trust and respect that can be summarised as 'I–thou'. This belief has gradually permeated all education in recent years, and recent research by Phillips *et al* (1994) advocates a strengthening of this approach:

> First, evidence is collected. Next, this is reflected upon by the student, the mentor and the lecturer. Because each of them interprets the evidence according to their own particular framework — or discourse — there is then a need for dialogue between the student . . . the mentor . . . and the lecturer. The dialogue allows separate interpretations to be discussed, learned from and integrated.

Students are future colleagues whose ability to self-assess needs to be nurtured. Whilst the need for one person to make a judgement of another's abilities will always mitigate against the formation of a truly equal partnership, this should be the optimum relationship for which all strive.

*Published forms of assessment such as standardised tests mould . . . curricula and inhibit new developments.*
It is certain that centrally set examinations constrain course development, and it is a source of relief (as well as anxiety for the monitoring of national

standards) that the question of content and form of assessments now features as an integral part of course design. The assessment of practice, however, raises some interesting questions in this respect. Knowles (1973) argues that adult learners should set their own objectives. Many nursing curricula, including the *Nursing Times* Open Learning (NTOL) conversion course, have based the assessment of practice on outcomes negotiated between student and teacher. NVQ competences are, on the other hand, predetermined. The extent to which these come to be felt as a constraint remains to be seen.

## The purpose of assessment

Having acknowledged the arguments against assessment, the reader may question why one assesses.

### To protect an innocent public

There have been many discussions in the literature on the nature of professions, but one key characteristic is the operation of control of access to the appropriate register, which is perceived as offering some measure of public protection. Bligh (1975) argues with justification that, on the contrary, professional examinations license individuals to do things that were not a feature of their training. This is manifestly true for even the most conservative of professions. Certainly completion of a pre-registration programme of nurse education does not confer all the knowledge and clinical skill that a newly qualified staff nurse may be required to demonstrate during a lifetime of employment. However the public have a fundamental entitlement to expect competence from the qualified nurse and protection against unsafe practice. The machinery of statutory registration is designed to ensure that those legally entitled to call themselves 'nurse' possess the competences described in the appropriate part of the Nurses, Midwives and Health Visitors Act 1983 and subsequent amendment (1987). However, qualifying and licensing procedures such as nurse registration share some of the characteristics and shortcomings of the driving test or the MOT certificate, i.e. the requirements of the test were satisfied at the time at which it was undergone, and obviously skills can decay or essential new skills remain undeveloped. The UKCC (1992) requires that the nurse must:

'maintain and improve professional knowledge and competence'.

However providing nurses with the appropriate resources and opportunities for retaining and developing their skills has been, until relatively recently, an area of gross neglect. The move towards the maintenance of a live register, linked to the Post-Registration Education and Practice (PREP) proposals for the need to demonstrate participation in development activities is further discussed in Chapter 7.

## To predict the future behaviour of nurses

The predictive validity of an assessment strategy is one of its most important purposes yet also the most difficult to achieve. When, at the point of selection, candidates have satisfied the selectors that they have the potential to successfully complete the programme of study, a prediction has been made. The rate of attrition in some nurse education programmes testifies to the unsatisfactory nature of these predictions in many cases.

Throughout a period of study, formative and summative assessments alike are made, which of themselves purport, whether implicitly or explicitly, to have predictive properties. Students are permitted to proceed to the next module or part of the course on the basis of successful completion of the former. Finally, an overall assessment has to be made that will permit the student to register as a nurse. Yet another prediction is made that as long as they remain registered practitioners, they will be competent. Whilst this is occasionally demonstrated not to be so (by the action of the professional conduct committee in removing names from the register), we have no such evidence of those who are judged unfit to practise. False negatives — those who have been wrongly judged not to possess the required competences — are lost to the profession for ever.

## To judge the level of student achievement

Throughout the programme of training it is essential that students should be aware of their level of achievement. Assessments that measure a broad range of achievement at the conclusion of the module or course are described as *summative*. Certainly a pass/fail decision will be made, and frequently grades are awarded. In contrast *formative* assessments are designed to give feedback to both student and teacher of progress towards the final goal. The emphasis in this category of assessment is on analysis of the strengths and weaknesses of students in order to guide them for the future. It is generally the practice not to grade this type of work, but it is interesting to note that students may press for grades to be given. This need for 'bottom line' information reflects the underlying anxieties of students about the assessment process and the power of examiners.

## To monitor student progress

It is necessary that both students and their teachers should be able to monitor the level of achievement as the course progresses. As previously described in Chapter 3 a knowledge of results as a re-reinforcement and reward is important in the learning process. A sequence of intermittent assessments enables the student's progress to be monitored. In isolation the assessment will reveal the student's location relative to his or her own personal learning objectives and the objectives of the specific module or unit of the course, but it also provides information on performance relative to that of other students. Monitoring individual and group performance enables the early detection of student learning difficulties and the implementation of appropriate remedial action.

In recent years it has been unfashionable, indeed often offensive, to legitimise the role of competition in education. There is no doubt that creating a ruthless climate of competition is damaging for all concerned; after all the prize of registration is accessible to all who have commenced training, at least in theory. However it has also to be acknowledged that much of man's ingenuity, creativity, inventiveness and productivity can be directly traced back to competitiveness. Whether students should be encouraged to compare their assessment results is a contentious issue. The reality is that, with or without our consent, our students compare their grades and marks, success and failure. It might be that promoting a climate of gentle competitiveness in assessment would be more honest than the fraudulent denial of the existence of the phenomenon.

*To motivate students*

It is self-evident that most students become increasingly conscientious about their studies in relation to assessed parts of the course. Examinations in particular appear to concentrate the mind. In the main this is healthy and desirable, although motivation for achievement and the perceived need to study should be a by-product of assessment and not one of its major purposes. The nature of a programme ought to have sufficient intrinsic worth to the individual that motivation comes from inside the student rather from the fear of failure. Ultimately if registered nurses are to be flexible practitioners engaged in learning for life, one of the outcomes for all courses of study should be the fostering of the individual's responsibility to clients. Delivering high quality care should be the motivator for learning.

In addition to their motivating effect, however, assignment deadlines and looming examinations are occasions for stress. Since 1963, when Still first demonstrated that the incidence of psychiatric referrals amongst university students increased as examinations approached, a steady stream of research has confirmed this to be the case. For some students stress is felt particularly keenly in relation to summative terminal examinations, and the introduction of continuous assessment often reduces stress levels. For others the introduction of continuous assessment has served merely to elongate the period of stress they experience.

*To measure the effectiveness of teaching*

It is not unreasonable to assume that the students' achievement, as measured by examination success, is in part related to the effectiveness of their teachers and mentors; indeed teachers appear readily to associate themselves with their students' success. Whilst success is an indicator of the effectiveness of teaching, this must be viewed in the context of assessment as rigorous quality control. It follows that where assessments are marked against specific criteria, fluctuations in examination results will inevitably occur, reflecting the ability of different student groups. However persistently poor performance by the students of one teacher in relation to those supported by other teachers is a legitimate cause for concern and should be placed alongside students' evaluations of the acceptabilility of that teacher's performance.

Whilst publicly at least it may appear that student failure is more likely to be perceived as being the fault of the student than of the teacher, there is evidence that both teachers and clinical mentors engage in a great deal of heart-searching when a student fails to reach the required standard.

### To assess competence

It is worth pausing to consider the concept of competence. Wood (1987) defines it thus:

'The ability to use knowledge, product and process skills and, as a result, act effectively to achieve a purpose.'

He goes on to make the following important distinction:

'Competence refers to what a person knows or can do under ideal circumstances, whereas performance refers to what is actually done in existing circumstances.'

Competence and performance do not necessarily correlate. A student may be competent to pass an examination but because of hay fever or pre-menstrual tension may fail to perform adequately on the day. Conversely, a student who is not competent in principles of microbiology and who consistently contaminates instruments during the performance of an aseptic technique may on some occasions, and entirely by accident, perform to an acceptable standard.

For Benner (1982) competence falls midway between the performance of the beginner (novice) and the unthinking smooth and adaptable performance of the 'expert'. It consists of conscious, deliberate planning, includes the accurate setting of priorities and exhibits smooth effective performance in routine situations. Competence contrasts to the novice's halting jerky behaviour, where every part of every movement is conscious (remember the first attempts at driving a car?), and the immense repertoire of instinctive behaviours exhibited by the expert who can draw on experience and respond even to major crises appropriately, effectively and efficiently. Girot (1993) described the attributes that characterise overall competence and non-competence in learner nurses.

The assessment of practice is of course the cornerstone of the NVQ framework. The principles of assessment of work-based learning espoused by the National Council for Vocational Qualifications are somewhat different from those traditionally in use in nurse education. Their influence has been great, as clinical assessors who have been required to meet the requirements of the National Standards for Assessment and Verification in their work with health care assistants will attest. The key features of NVQ assessment are as follows:

— *Assessment, not teaching, is the cornerstone.* Once individuals have demonstrated competence in any area, both in terms of knowledge and practice, they are deemed to have completed the unit, whether the period of studentship is one week or six months. This is radically different from the concept of nurse education where the period of study is set out in statute.
— *Reliability is sought by a system of internal and external assessors* who review the evidence and the judgement of the assessor. This formalises the traditional requirement in nurse education that all members of the team should be involved in the assessment process.
— *Assessment centres around the collection of evidence,* the onus for which is on the student. Thus nurses might appear before their assessors armed with care plans written for their patients, records of care delivered, records of meetings that they chaired or in which they participated, or witness statements as to their competence. This compilation of a variety of assessment evidence is recommended for adoption by the profession by Phillips *et al* (1994).
— *Assessors are trained to national standards,* published by the Training and Development Lead Body. For example one of the elements for the unit 'assess candidate performance' is 'collect and judge performance evidence against criteria'. The performance criteria that assessors have to meet in order to show competence in that area are as follows:

  (i) The candidate is encouraged to identify and present relevant evidence.
 (ii) Candidate performance is accurately assessed against elements and performance criteria.
(iii) Only the specified performance criteria are used in assessments.
 (iv) The evidence can be attributed to the candidate.
  (v) Any preset simulations and tests are correctly administered.
 (vi) The assessor is as unobtrusive as is practicable whilst observing the candidate.
(vii) Difficulties in interpreting performance criteria are referred promptly to the appropriate authority.

## Assessment strategy

In the past 30 years we have witnessed a profound change in attitudes to assessment. Clearly there have been innovations in assessment methods, but more fundamentally there has been a major conceptual shift, some components of which are highlighted in Fig. 5.1.

Perhaps the most important is the change in the relationship between teachers and students. In many programmes of study students define their own learning objectives and engage in contracting processes to determine the learning resources upon which they will draw in order to meet those needs. It has been recognised that self-assessment is a fundamental component of reflective practice and is therefore a skill that should be fostered in its own right. With the development of Project 2000 diploma courses, there has been a tendency to move away from the descriptions of practice that were so much a feature of traditional training and in particular of the final determinate examination. Increasingly, whilst application to practice remains an important criterion, the depth of theory underpinning practice requires to be tested in its own right. A sound understanding of the '-ologies' and how they inform the practice of nursing is important, but their significance is only realised in the care setting. For too long practical assessors have perceived their role as being less important than that of those who mark examination papers, and it is incumbent upon those who have a responsibility for education to take steps to support assessors in the making of professional judgements. At the same time assessors must accept that putting the assessment of practice in the centre of the process brings with it increased scrutiny. As examination papers are marked by more than one teacher and then subsequently marked by external examiners, so future assessors of practice must come to accept the practice of offering a rationale for their judgements to a verifier or external examiner as part of a natural process of justice rather than, as now, a threatening intrusion into private mental processes.

The detailed identification and analysis of educational objectives into cognitive, affective and psychomotor categories undertaken by Bloom and his associates was discussed in Chapter 3. Scrutiny of nursing curricula reveals that this tripartite structuring of human abilities is much favoured by nurse and indeed general educationalists. Course objectives are frequently presented under the distinct headings of knowledge, attitudes and skills. However when it comes to assessment, methods of determining achievement in the cognitive (knowledge) domain appear to have been far more extensively developed than those in the

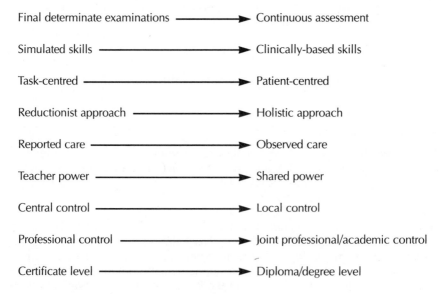

| | |
|---|---|
| Final determinate examinations | Continuous assessment |
| Simulated skills | Clinically-based skills |
| Task-centred | Patient-centred |
| Reductionist approach | Holistic approach |
| Reported care | Observed care |
| Teacher power | Shared power |
| Central control | Local control |
| Professional control | Joint professional/academic control |
| Certificate level | Diploma/degree level |

Fig. 5.1    Dimensional changes in assessment

affective (attitudes) or psychomotor (skills) categories. Assessment grids and marking schemes that employ a cognitive taxonomy are relatively common, but those relating to the affective and psychomotor domain were conspicuous by their absence. The view might be expressed that these have at least in part been addressed by the publication of NVQ standards, including those of the 'value based units', but these are presented as pragmatic assessment instruments rather than as taxonomies based on any identifiable learning theory. Concentration on Bloom has meant that there has been a potential for cognition, or theory, to dominate assessment, as argued above. This has been compounded by the almost inevitable need to promote the academic content of the first diploma courses in order to render them acceptable to the universities, many of whom found nursing a strange entity with which to deal. Since the publication of the first edition of this book, much interest has been shown in the use of the holistic experiential approach to curriculum design. Steinaker & Bell (1979) identify specific assessment techniques that they recommend should be employed at each level of their taxonomy (Fig. 5.2).

In addition to this 'whole student' perspective of assessment, such an approach ensures that the assessment techniques are compatible with the abilities being measured. Further, and significantly, assessment is congruent with the other components of curricular activity, and in this respect domination of the curriculum by assessment is averted. It should also be noted that student self-assessment is an explicit requirement of the taxonomy and is consistent with the androgogical approach discussed earlier in this chapter. In relation to the 'teacher-domination–student-participation' dimension, there has been a

| | |
|---|---|
| Exposure | Observing student reaction to the initial activities to determine attention; understanding of terms, scenes and purpose; and readiness/willingness to proceed. |
| Participation | Examining student choices; signals of understanding or of lack of understanding; replications; discussions; questioning to determine understanding; ability to succeed; and, where appropriate, explanation of how the learner 'would do it' if given the opportunity. |
| Identification | Using criteria, teacher-developed tests or assignments and mental or actual checklists to assess student progress and teaching or unit effectiveness. |
| Internalisation | Using projective measures such as open-ended anonymous response questionnaires and/or direct measures such as rating scales and interviews; using a post- and re-test method in which a different test form or assignment is given at a later date and is compared with the original test or assignment to determine retention. |
| Dissemination | Using student self-assessment instruments; assessing the time devoted to tasks, the variety of techniques employed to use or to promote the learning and/or the degree of influence achieved. |

Fig. 5.2 The experiential taxonomy

considerable move towards student self-assessment, a move thoroughly consistent with the need to produce flexible practitioners, engaged in a future of lifelong learning — a being for whom employers are currently devoutly seeking. The means by which such a person may be identified are discussed in Chapter 6.

## References

Benner P (1984) *From Novice to Expert: Excellence and Power in Clinical Nursing Practice.* California: Addison Wesley

Bligh D (1975) *Teaching Students.* Exeter: UETS

Broadfoot P (1986) *Profiles and Records of Achievement.* London: Cassell

DHSS (1983) *The Nurses, Midwives and Health Visitors Rules Approval Order 1983* (Cmnd 873). London: HMSO

Girot E A (1993) Assessment of competence in clinical practice — a phenomenological approach. *Journal of Advanced Nursing,* **18**: 114–19

Knowles M (1973) *The Adult Learner — A Neglected Species.* Houston: Gulf Publishing

Lankshear A J (1990) *Double Vision? A Comparative Study of the Attitudes of Teachers and Clinical Assessors to the Assessment of Student Nurses.* Unpublished thesis, University of York

Manpower Services Commission (1986) *Working Together, Education and Training.* London: Department of Employment

Miller C & Parlett M (1974) *Up to the Mark: A Study of the Examination Game.* London: SRHE

Minton D (1984) Evaluation and assessment in continuing. In *Teaching Strategies for Continuing Education.* London: City and Guilds Institute.

Phillips T, Shostack J, Bedford H and Robinson J (1994) *Assessment of Competence in Nursing and Midwifery Education (Project 2000). Final Report of the ACE Project.* Sheffield: ENB

Rowntree D (1987) *Assessing Students: How Shall We Know Them?* London: Kogan Page

Satterly D (1981) *Assessment in Schools.* Oxford: Basil Blackwell

Sims (1976) The critical incident technique in evaluating student nurse performance. *International Journal of Nursing Studies,* **13**: 123–30.

Steinaker N W & Bell M P (1979) *The Experiential Taxonomy: A New Approach to Teaching and Learning.* New York: Academic Press

Still R J (1963) *Psychological Illness among Students in the Examination Period.* Leeds: University of Leeds

UKCC (1986) *Project 2000 — A New Preparation for Practice.* London: UKCC

UKCC (1992) *Code of Professional Conduct.* London: UKCC

Wood R (1987) *Measurement and Assessment in Education and Psychology.* London: The Falmer Press

# 6
# Methods of Assessment

Continuous assessment became compulsory for all ENB-approved assessed courses in January 1990. In prospect it was a change to be welcomed. The previous edition of this book set out the case:

'The impetus for continuous assessment can be directly attributable to the patent injustice of 'one-off' final and determinate examinations where the competence demonstrated on the day may not be representative of the abilities demonstrated by the student throughout the course, where factors such as luck or anxiety may unfairly influence her performance. In practice, the use of a broader range of assessment techniques, more frequent assessment of student progress and achievement and the involvement of more individual assessors all conspire to dilute the deficiencies of traditional 'one-off' examinations. However, continuous assessment brings with it its own problems.'

Not least of these is its definition. Continuous assessment (also known as intermittent, regular or cumulative assessment) is variously interpreted in colleges and universities throughout the land, and indeed its working has been altered in the move to modularisation of courses.

Most systems of continuous assessment allow for the concept of compensation. This means that within a module, a poor result in one assignment or examination may be balanced by a better result given for a different piece of work. This, in theory at least, does not penalise students for one-off failures attributable to unrelated contextual factors. In nursing however there is a challenge that arises from the fact that, in relation to pre-registration education, the learning outcomes are statutorily defined. Compensation must be treated with extreme caution and, according to the Regulations of the ENB (1993), cannot be applied:

'when the examination failed:
   a forms a substantial proportion of the total assessment process
   b is central to the fulfilment of the course objectives
   c is testing an area of knowledge/competence required to be tested under the Nurses, Midwives and Health Visitors Rules, and which has not and will not be sufficiently tested elsewhere in the course

As it is difficult to conceive of a rationale for the inclusion of an assessment that fulfils none of the above criteria, the scope for compensation in pre-registration nursing courses is minimal. Thus a fail grade in one assessment cannot normally be balanced by a good pass in another. This sets continuous assessment in nursing apart from many systems in use.

Indeed in order to introduce continuous assessment at all, the UKCC had to issue 'Interpretative Principles' in order to overcome the fact that the requirement for a final written examination was enshrined in statute. These assumed that the final examination was to be conceived of as consisting of parts and that each element of a continuous assessment strategy was part of the final examination.

In reality, Rowntree (1987) argues, the issue is not one of continuous assessment (versus terminal assessment) but of continuous grading. The progress of students on courses has always been assessed throughout the course, but the issue is whether success in these components counts towards a final result or grading. With the advent of modularisation, assessments become linked to specific modules, which much be passed in order that the student be attributed with the credits attached to that module. Continuous assessment of modules may or may not be linked to a final whole year or whole course examination.

## Consideration of assessment methods

Assessments are tools that give students opportunities to demonstrate the learning that has taken place. As with research methods, each has its strengths and weaknesses, and a sound assessment strategy will utilise a number of methods in order to receive a comprehensive picture of the student. It should be clearly understood that continuous assessment does not preclude examinations, and indeed it is a requirement laid down by the ENB that at least one unseen examination should figure in each pre-registration course. The reasons for this are discussed later in this chapter. As to the amount of assessment to be completed in total, a wide variation in requirements can be traced across the country. Some universities have a rule of thumb that each module of ten credits should be assessed by 3000 written words. A pre-registration diploma course of 240 credits could therefore demand that the student write 72 000 words. Some universities will allow a reduction against the assessment of practice, but there is little consistency across the country, with the exception of those new universities that still adhere to the guidelines of the late Council for National Academic Awards and which do, at the time of writing, offer a more or less unified approach.

As assessment strategies can be described in relation to a number of continua (see Chapter 5), so can methods. A consideration of the following dimensions may be useful:

subjective–objective
convergent–divergent
valid–invalid
reliable–unreliable
practical–theoretical
insular–collaborative
humanistic–behavioural

## Subjective–objective

The earlier edition of this book pointed out that, at the time of writing, methods of assessment in use in colleges and schools of nursing were predominantly objective, i.e. assessed by a person or people other than the student. As has been seen in Chapter 5, there has been, since this was written, a fundamental shift in relation to this dimension. Demands from employers for an increasingly flexible group of professionals, coupled with demands from universities to demonstrate the use of higher cognitive processes in the practice setting, led to a burgeoning interest in the work of Schön (1980). Schön argues that in order to equip professionals to deal with decision-making in a lifetime of complex and unique encounters, their education should centre around the principles of reflection-in-action. That means that students should base their studies around the experience of practice, learning to recall salient episodes, analyse them, criticise the actions and decisions taken within the context of the unique occurrence, and offer considered alternative strategies that might have been deployed. It implies that learning, and the assessment of that learning, should be firmly based in the complex messiness of the practical setting and that principles for action should be formulated and articulated by the student on the basis of experience. Students learn to be self-critical, continuously reviewing their practice and considering alternative strategies for improvement in the quality of service given to clients — hence the movement away from objective to subjective methods. Students are encouraged to keep reflective diaries and record critical incidents as a means of preserving and analysing their contribution to practice. These methods are often poorly understood by students, and clinical assessors have a key role to play in encouraging their diligent use. These approaches keep assessment real, based as they are in the messy confusion that is everyday life in the nursing care of patients and clients.

## Convergent–divergent

Like convergent lines, which eventually meet regardless of their distance from each other at the start, convergent tests are those in which all students could be expected to produce the same answer to a question regardless of experience or reading. The ultimate convergent test is the multiple choice question, closely followed by short answer questions which require factual answers. These tests, easy to mark, are useful in testing the recall of knowledge, the understanding of relationships and the ability to analyse.

Divergent assessments, on the other hand, assume that students will follow their own areas of interest and will produce at the end of the period widely differing pieces of work. Projects and research studies are typical examples of divergent work. Whilst these allow students to develop arguments, solve problems, synthesise material and examine their own views in relation to those of others, they can give rise to considerable problems in marking. It clearly becomes impossible for examiners to preordain the scope of the content. Instead typical marking criteria focus on the extent and use of available literature, the clarity and logical development of the argument, the application of theory to practice, the way in which the work is structured and organised and the degree of reflection shown.

## Valid–invalid

Assessments should measure what they purport to measure — in other words, they should be valid. Whilst this appears to be a requirement so fundamental as to be hardly worth stating, the reality is that validity is extremely difficult to demonstrate. As an illustration Rowntree (1987) tells of an experience of his own, when as a young student he stood outside the door of an examination room clutching a piece of paper on which were written the mathematics formulae, the knowledge of which was fundamental to the examination. When the students were admitted to the room, he screwed up the piece of paper and ran to his desk, whereupon he reproduced the formulae on a piece of 'rough' paper provided. Whatever abilities the examiners believed they were testing, it was presumably not the ability to retain an image for a 20-second dash across a room. Wood (1987) makes the following point:

> 'a test cannot be valid in general, it is valid for a purpose. Depending on purpose, the validity of an A level examination can be assessed primarily either in terms of its soundness as a test of achievement (syllabus coverage) or its value for predicting suitability for a university. Likewise a test can be valid and not valid, as for example an A level examination that predicts university success for women but not for men. Context matters crucially.'

| | |
|---|---|
| Predictive validity | Extent to which the test accurately predicts a future event, such as successful completion of the whole course. |
| Content validity | Extent to which the test samples all of the relevant curriculum content. |
| Face validity | Extent to which a test appears to be relevant. |
| Construct validity | Degree to which a test measures an abstract concept (like caring). |
| Inter-rater reliability | More than one marker or assessor agrees on the outcome in respect of any one student. |
| Test–retest reliability | If administered on another occasion, the outcome in respect of each student is the same. |

Fig. 6.1 Types of validity and reliability

There is therefore no point in asking *whether* a test is valid, but rather *to what extent* it is valid and in what circumstances. The validity of an assessment has a number of dimensions (Fig. 6.1). Examinations should look right! For example, the use of a written test to assess the students' ability to receive and admit a patient into hospital may reveal that they understand the principles but will not confirm that they possess the complex array of observational, analytical and technical skills required. A written test in this example would lack face validity. Additionally an assessment strategy should show content validity. This is defined by Kempa (1986) as the 'extent to which a test or examination samples the content and/or the range of objectives of the course or curriculum to which it relates'. In other words all parts of the course should be assessed. Additionally a test should have concurrent validity — the 'extent to which scores derived from a test relate to scores obtained on an external criterion', i.e. the correlation between scores on tests that are measuring the same outcomes.

It is an axiomatic but nevertheless surprising statement that the only really valid way to test nursing ability is in the practice setting. Where underpinning theory is being examined, the assessment should relate to the practice setting. A word of warning however: most of the readers of this book will well remember the traditional format of final examination papers which gave a pen-picture of a patient or client and asked candidates to describe the nursing care. In a seminal but embarrassing (for the establishment) piece of work, Bendall, as long ago as 1975, demonstrated that what nurses said they would do in an examination paper of this sort did not match with what they actually did in practice. Whilst the statistical basis of Bendall's work was later challenged (Hutchings 1981), experience tends to uphold the findings. Face validity can lull us into a false sense of security. Some assessments may appear more valid than others. A statistics test using nursing research examples will appear more valid than one using examples from other types of research, yet this difference is merely cosmetic. The skills tested are the same in both cases.

Validity is an important principle that must be considered at every stage but, like the notion of quality, is a slippery concept. There is at the moment a raging debate on the depth of teaching of the biological sciences in nursing. Many university lecturers in the subject are appalled by the depth to which the subject is taught (and assessed) in nursing. Yet to what depth do nurses need to know about the structure and functioning of the body? When was the last time knowledge of the structure of Peyer's Patches actively informed someone's nursing care? Yet patients ask profound and perceptive questions about their symptoms, and a superficial knowledge will soon be found wanting. Validity is an issue for teaching as well as assessing.

## Reliable–unreliable

Reliability refers to the extent to which results can be reproduced and is a major issue when practical assessment strategies are discussed. How can an assurance be given that the same situation will be perceived in the same way by two different assessors or by the same assessor on two different occasions?

Written work can at least be marked, re-marked, moderated and appealed against. Throughout the process of consideration, and regardless of how many people judge over a period of time, the work stays constant. In the practical situation however, unless recourse is taken to complex and inherently distracting technology, a unique and complex situation lives on only in the memories of assessor and assessed. As Harrison (1984) argues, 'Assessment of performance, as opposed to that of knowledge, poses formidable problems about how it is to be judged fairly'.

Returning to the section above dealing with subjectivity and objectivity, the same arguments apply. By and large objectivity is seen to be reliable and subjectivity unreliable. Increasing reliability in the practice setting involves using minutely defined performance criteria that leave no room for deviation on the part of assessors and in some areas of activity are perfectly possible. Detailed performance criteria for bathing a patient could include defining the depth and temperature of the water and describing the preparation of the patient. At the expense of voluminous practical assessment documents, it is possible to increase reliability in terms of what is demonstrated. As soon as the focus shifts to the manner in which care is carried out, the problems commence. To continue the example above, a performance criterion such as 'ensures the dignity of the patient at all times' will be open to various interpretations, from those who think that the patient's dignity is preserved so long as the bathroom door is closed to those who will drape the patient's genitals with a towel until he or she is submerged beneath the water. In reality such a statement is patient dependent. One person's dignity will be offended by behaviour vital to the dignity of another. Such meticulous descriptions of performance may increase reliability but they do not necessarily improve individually designed programmes of care.

These are not problems confined to nursing, and the profession should congratulate itself on the ongoing debate around the assessment of practice. Whilst Kelly (1955) argued that the concept of reliability and validity were 'sacred cows' that denied both changing situations and the value and reality of individual perception, they remain important absolutes against which real life assessments will be measured.

### Practical–theoretical

This may at first sight be less of a continuum and more of a simple distinction between two types of assessment: practical assessment is the judgement of the ability to perform; theoretical assessment is a judgement of the ability to represent in words the possession of knowledge, attitudes and skills. Yet in reality the distinction is not so clear. Compare for example the student sitting a viva voce examination and the student discussing with a practical assessor the occasions on which he or she has had an opportunity to demonstrate some ability that the assessor has not directly observed. The two conversations might look the same, yet the results of one discussion would be recorded within the documentation relating to theoretical assessment and the other in practical assessment papers. Consider too the old classroom practical tests set by the General Nursing Council some years ago, in which students had to demonstrate procedures and skills under controlled conditions. This was a test of practical ability, i.e. of skill and understanding of the principles underpinning the skill, but might arguably be said to be rather further removed from the complex reality of life than for example a good care study.

Incidentally this notion of testing skill out of context, thought by many to be outdated, may reappear in the next decade as NHS Trusts, struggling with the need to establish the most cost-effective skill mix patterns, make demands on colleges and departments of nursing to equip students with basic skills before placement allocations commence. This de-contextualised testing of skill *in the early stages of its acquisition* makes sense. None of us learned clutch control on the High Street, and, as Dreyfus & Dreyfus (1980) remind us, airlines invest in phenomenally expensive flight simulators to test pilot skill before giving them charge of immeasurably more expensive aircraft full of passengers. There is no added educational value in having a patient collapse whilst a student nurse connects up suction apparatus for the first time. Such simulations are widely used in the USA and go hand in hand with the assessment of that skill in patient areas.

Much has been said in this book so far of the centrality and importance of the assessment of nursing practice. The tools in use for so doing vary in their approach and are universally flawed. Firstly, there is a tendency towards generalising skills so that significant but discrete levels of attainment are concealed. Further, in many documents, each of the dimensions may be weighted equally, although in reality some skills may be more significant or important than others. In some documents a student who is industrious, prompt, well-groomed and courteous could pass overall despite failing on some other key dimensions. Ready-written profiling documents frequently confuse a number of elements, so that in reality a student may straddle two or three descriptive boxes (Fig. 6.2).

In assessing the complex array of skills required, a variety of techniques must be used. At best, individual assessments are a little like taking snapshots — the picture reveals precisely what was happening at the instant the film was exposed. Consequently the more snaps that are taken, the greater the overall impression and understanding of the subject. There is also a case for passing the camera around as different individuals may wish to focus on alternative aspects of the subject. To develop this analogy further, it may well be that some of our shots will be out of focus, but as long as this is realised, important though restricted information will still be available. What is being advocated here is the need for a comprehensive portrayal of student abilities. Phillips *et al* (1994) recommend that 'assessment documentation should be broadened to include evidence contributed by more than one accredited witness and used as the basis of dialogue about knowledge skills understanding and attitudes'.

| Inadequate records kept | Record-keeping minimal or inaccurate | Records generally accurate but unclear or sketchy | Records usually accurate and informative | Records always clear concise and accurate |
|---|---|---|---|---|
| | | | | |

Fig. 6.2 Profiling statements confusing multiple factors

*Insular–collaborative*

Assessment methods can be designed to ensure that the student works alone; the most effective tool in this respect being the examination. In traditional examinations desks are spaced to prevent contact between candidates, talking is forbidden and invigilators patrol the floor to ensure that the rules are followed. This scenario is so familiar to us all that we scarcely question it, yet the validity of such an environment must be questioned. In what situations occurring in life would we ever find ourselves so totally divorced from our fellow man? Yet if all work was collaborative, how could we be sure that the candidate applying for entry to the Register was competent in his or her own right? Truly the strength of the examination as a method is that it is the only situation in which the writer is observed to write that which is later judged. Various forms of the examination have been introduced into the lexicon in recent years. The Open Book Examination, in which permission is given to carry books into the examination, allows candidates to collaborate with the minds of writers but simultaneously establishes that he or she has the ability to access these sources. Other variants of the examination are discussed at the end of this chapter.

Collaborative working can be encouraged in relation to community profiles, projects, research studies and, inevitably, in the practical setting. The students' ability to relate to peers thus becomes an integral part of the assessment. Compare the 'exposure on a mountain' type of management assessment exercise where the ability to motivate/lead or work with a team is assessed under trying conditions. There are of course difficulties in ensuring that each student has contributed equally to the process of compiling a successful submission or in determining the reason for failure. Yet these should not deter us from their use. In real life managers fail as a result of their subordinates' failures — and the reverse is also the case. We are all dependent on each other's work, and early exposure to the reality of this could be argued to be a preparation for life.

*Humanistic–behavioural*

Attempts have been made to render assessment, particularly in relation to practice, more reliable by the use of clearly observed and defined behaviours. Whilst the motives for this approach are both understandable and laudable, the results are frequently nonsensical. At best, the tendency is to measure that which is measurable rather than that which is important.

A recent attempt to utilise behavioural objectives in the assessment of student nurses floundered on the grounds of impracticality, as Collingwood (1990) found. The author's own experience illustrates the invalid nature of one attempt to break down a complex activity (communication) into component parts and to state the number of times the student had to demonstrate each of the elements. This, we were assured, would ensure fairness as each student would know precisely what he had to do in order to pass the assessment. So it proved. One student complied precisely with the requirements and was duly passed on this aspect of the assessment. Subsequently the trained staff of the ward, who had been involved in his assessment, took up their pens and wrote a damning description of his communication skills, which had on numerous occasions left patients in tears and colleagues speechless! Personal attributes such as a caring manner and the degree of interest in their patients and their work are, in the view of many assessors, amongst the most important qualities of student nurses. Whilst behavioural cues that indicate the possession of these qualities can be isolated, they can never define them entirely. Ironically when an attribute is difficult to describe in behavioural terms, it is tempting to adopt the line of least resistance and remove it from the assessment document entirely.

## The preparation and role of assessors

At the time of writing the intention is that assessors of student nurses and midwives will have been prepared by means of completion of the ENB 997/998 Teaching and Assessing in Midwifery/Nursing Practice course. In reality a substantial number of those involved in assessment have had a considerably shorter preparation through completion of an Art of Examining course or as part of Project 2000 staff preparation. Increasingly assessors are being trained to the standards of the Training and Development Lead Body of the National Council for Vocational Qualifications, which were discussed in Chapter 5.

## Others involved in the assessment process

### The student

Most systems of practical assessment and many theoretical assessments contain opportunities for students to self-assess. This process of self-assessment is said to assist in motivating students by encouraging them to work to their own standards rather than those of others. This in turn, according to Ramsden (1985), gives rise to in-depth rather than superficial approaches to learning. Students are required to grade their own assignments or critically assess their achievement of practice outcomes. This assessment then has to be compared against that of the assigned assessor and a negotiated grade given. But can students reasonably be trusted to make an honest assessment of their work when they have such a vested interest in the outcome? The assumption is often made that students will tend to over-estimate their performance, but a variety of studies (Bligh 1975, Falchicoff 1986) have indicated that this is not in fact the case.

Counselling is often considered as exclusively a technique for helping a student with a problem situation. However client-centred problem-solving models of counselling demand goal-setting and problem-solving based on principles of self-assessment. In this context counselling is a particularly useful method of helping the student to make an insightful assessment of his or her own ability. Role construct repertory tests and grids derived from personal construct psychology (Kelly 1955) have been used as a method of self-assessment in teacher training (Pope 1978). A nursing application of repertory grids was described by Nicklin (1984). McHale (1985) describes a variety of techniques, including psychometric tests, video feedback and personal and group analysis by an assessor trained in the technique of self-awareness assessment. Learning logs and records of achievement are a useful device for students to capture information about their learning experiences. Subsequent reflection and analysis provide an opportunity for personal assessment of progress that can be compared with the impressions and opinions of supervisors, teachers and peers.

### Peer assessment

The student's peers have a significant contribution to make in the overall assessment process, and peer review and peer audit are increasingly features of professional practice. Peer assessment during training provides opportunities for students to rate each other's work. It enlarges the process of reflection to allow students to analyse the work of others and to give honest but sympathetic feedback. The fact that peers work for sustained periods in close proximity inevitably means they have the opportunity to make assessments that are inaccessible to others. It is challenging, difficult to do, time consuming and vital in preparing aspiring professionals to evaluate the work of others. It also gives insight into the difficulties inherent in the process and enables the development of empathy between students and those charged with the formation of final judgements.

### Patient/client assessment

As recipients of the care delivered by students, patients and clients are a legitimate source of assessment data, but formalising and gaining access to the assessments that patients are most certainly making is fraught with ethical and practical problems. There is however potential in considering and further developing the many quality audit documents currently in use as a source of information about the performance of individual staff. Patient comment and complaints facilities could and should feed into the assessment process for individual students.

## Profiling

In recent years there has been increasing emphasis on the value of profiling as a means of recording both formal study undertaken and that work-based learning which has been achieved without necessarily being formally organised or recognised. This is often discussed in relation to the Accreditation of Prior Experiential Learning (APEL), which is the mechanism by which informal learning (learning on-the-job or 'in the university of life') is judged in terms of academic worth. The concept of profiling puts students rather than courses, assessments or examinations, in the limelight and invites individuals to lay out evidence to demonstrate their learning. The process involves systematic analysis of the knowledge, skills and attitudes that an individual demonstrates in the workplace. The subsequent accumulation of evidence in support of the claim is the route to accreditation. In the introduction to the ENB's (1991) *Professional Portfolio*, it is said that:

'It is a way for you . . . to consider experiences in your professional and personal life and to evaluate the contribution those experiences make to your development and to improvements in client care.'

The strengths of profiling lie in the catholic nature of acceptable evidence and in the fact that relevance to the workplace is assured. There is no sense of artificiality as people pull together records of care, of contributions to meetings, witness statements, letters or proposals for change in order to demonstrate achievement. A student may be awarded a certain number of *general* credit points for a completed portfolio. If the portfolio is to be used towards a specific award, evidence must be set against the particular outcomes of the relevant programme. The resultant credit is termed '*specific* credit'. For the ENB Higher Award, students have to use their portfolios to demonstrate the achievement of 10 key characteristics (Fig. 6.3).

### Accountability

Expert Practitioners should have the ability to exercise professional accountability and responsibility, reflected in the degree to which they use professional skills, knowledge and expertise in changing environments, across professional boundaries, and in unfamiliar situations.

### Clinical Skills

Expert Practitioners should have specialist skills, knowledge and expertise in the practice area in which they are working, including a deeper and broader understanding of client/patient health needs, within the context of changing health care provision.

### Use of Research

Expert Practitioners should have the ability to use research enquiry and scholarship to plan, implement and evaluate concepts and strategies leading to improvements in care.

### Team Work

Expert Practitioners should have skills in team working, including multi-professional team working in which the leadership role changes in response to changing client needs, team leadership and team building skills to organise the delivery of care.

### Innovation

Expert Practitioners should have the ability to develop and use flexible and innovative approaches to practice that are appropriate to the needs of their client/patient or group, and are in line with the goals of the health service, and the employing authority.

### Health Promotion

Expert Practitioners should understand and use health promotion and preventative policies and strategies to achieve service targets.

### Staff Development

Expert Practitioners should have the ability to facilitate and assess the professional and other development of staff for whom they are responsible, and to act as a role model of professional practice.

**Resource Management**
Expert Practitioners should have the ability to take informed decisions about the allocation of resources for the benefit of individual clients and the client group with whom they are working.

**Quality of Care**
Expert Practitioners should have the ability to evaluate the quality of care delivered as an ongoing and cumulative process.

**Management of Change**
Expert Practitioners should have the ability to facilitate, initiate, manage and evaluate change in practice to improve quality of care.

Fig. 6.3    The ENB's ten key characteristics

## Making the final judgement

Decisions on whether students have achieved the standard required for a particular grade can be made in two ways.

### Criterion referenced assessment

This measures a student's skills and abilities against predetermined criteria. The issue here for the assessor is quite clear: whether or not the student has demonstrated the criteria required by this particular assessment. However there are inherent difficulties in deciding the degree of specificity required. The NVQ performance criteria for health care assistants uses tightly defined statements that can be used as a checklist, yet even in this nationally devised strategy, the criteria for the value based units require subjective judgements to be made.

Nursing is both an art and a science, and whilst the latter is amenable to reduction to criteria, the former tends to be less so. On what clear criteria is Beethoven's Ninth (Choral) Symphony judged as great music? As the constructs to be tested become more complex, the emphasis is increasingly on broadly based outcomes. 'Caring', 'creativity' or 'reflective practice' cannot be measured against behavioural outcomes, although the concepts can be unpacked so that there is some agreement between assessors on what it is they are looking for.

### Norm referenced assessment

Mobley *et al* (1986) describe this approach as 'a system in which a predetermined proportion of the candidates are allocated to each of the grades regardless of the quality of the work produced by the candidate. Hence the grade awarded to a candidate depends not only on his or her performance, but also on the performance of other candidates entered for the same examination'. In other words, before the examination is taken, it is declared that the top 5% will receive an A grade, the next 10% a B and so on. This is the basis on which A levels are still awarded, although the old norm referenced O levels have given way to criterion referenced GCSEs. Whilst many would argue that this system is unfair — some would say iniquitously so — most people carry around an expectation of consistency of pass rates. If a programme of study carries a normal pass rate of 86%, questions are likely to be asked if, on one occasion, this drops to 50%. Assessors feel exceedingly uncomfortable if they are at any one time dealing with a decision to fail two or more students on placement in their area (Lankshear 1990).

In reality criteria and their interpretation are informed by expectations based on normative observations. Additionally these normative criteria, used implicitly rather than explicitly, act as a check on the requirements of examinations and assessments, to the extent that a consistent pass rate of 20% in a theoretical examination will raise questions as to the appropriateness of that examination for the students at that time. Educationalists should be warned that changing an assessment for those reasons will be described as a cynical moving of the goalposts in order to improve the institution's performance indicators!

Hepworth (1989) comments on the anxiety and defensiveness that the subject of professional judgement raised in both students and assessors, particularly if that judgement is challenged or if it is suggested that the process should be examined. Many assessors so challenged felt that their decision should be good enough. Yet the term cannot be used, as it frequently appears to be, like a crucifix to throw in the face of the devil of enquiry. The assessment of students is a judgement based on cues, just as a doctor's diagnosis is based on the interpretation of signs and symptoms. Dowie's review of the decision-making process in medicine offers a lens diagram that can be readily adapted to illustrate the task (Fig. 6.4).

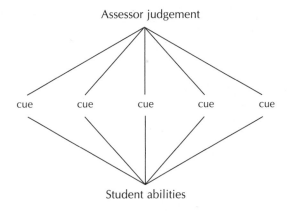

Fig. 6.4    Lens diagram

Table 6.1 Summary of advantages and disadvantages of non-clinical assessment methods

| Method | Advantages | Disadvantages |
|---|---|---|
| **Timed unseen examination** | Work known to be that of candidate. Evidence of ability to work under time pressure. All students sit same paper. | Favour students who study the process of examinations to 'question spot' and beat the system. Take place on one day and results are affected by individual health problems and short-term worries that would not contaminate longer studies. Where a choice of questions exists, students through individual combinations of questions in effect sit different papers. |
| **Seen examination** | Area of revision is defined so activity is focused and greater depth of knowledge can be expected. | Reduced coverage of the syllabus; students not motivated to learn what is not going to be tested. |
| **Open book examination** | Students do not have to memorise small facts. Demonstration of familiarity with key texts in such a way that pertinent information can be accessed quickly under pressure. | Facilitates cheating as students are permitted to carry materials into the room. No guarantee that students have any knowledge in their memory banks. |
| **Short answer tests** | Assessment of knowledge of information. Good coverage of a subject. Good inter-marker reliability. | Limited scope to demonstrate creativity, originality and problem-solving skills. |

| Method | | |
|---|---|---|
| **Objective tests** | Comprehensive syllabus coverage. 'Absolute' marking criteria. Permits compilation of a bank of researched questions. Easy to mark. Can be self-administered. | Construction of valid items notoriously difficult. Permits guessing. Right or wrong marking does not reflect many situations and is antithetical to the concept of individualised care. |
| **Care studies** | Permit integration of theory and practice. Students are required to examine critically the care prescribed and given. Integrate knowledge drawn from a variety of subject specialisms. | May reflect idealised standards of care rather than care given. Increasingly difficult to arrange as patient stays get shorter. |
| **Projects/research-based assignments** | Skills of active enquiry, information testing, hypothesis testing, problem-solving and critical analysis. Students can choose areas of study that reflect their own interests. | Notoriously difficult to grade students fairly in relation to one another as subjects may require different approaches. Extent of available existing literature also leads to inequity. |
| **Simulations** | Assessments of specific skills where patient safety is not compromised. | Ignores complexity of environment. |
| **Viva voce examinations** | Assessment of presentation and interpersonal skills, reasoning and debating abilities. | Favours students with good verbal ability. Difficult to conduct fairly. |

As doctors have had to come to terms with the difficulties of diagnostic deduction, so it must be accepted that assessment is a similarly inexact science in which differences of opinion will occasionally exist between honest professionals. An invitation to explain why a decision was reached in respect of an individual student is a legitimate request, yet assessors should be asked to explain the decision to pass a student at least as often as being asked why a fail grade was given. If an assessor is only ever asked to rationalise decisions to fail, the inevitable result is that assessors will avoid awarding such grades because of the 'hassle factor'. This leads to a vicious circle in which there is a 'failure to fail' students who do not reach the required standard (Lankshear 1990).

Methods of assessment as summarised in Table 6.1 have their strengths and weaknesses; there is no one perfect assessment tool. Much criticism of assessment is essentially a criticism of abuse of application or of interpretation. No assessment tool is faultless in its ability to differentiate those who give good nursing care from those who cannot. Assessments are aids to diagnosis and, like the stethoscope, the X-ray and the CAT scan, yield information that must be interpreted. Similarly, as a CAT scan will not reveal septicaemia nor an X-ray cirrhosis, it must be recognised so in educational assessment that all assessment tools have their limitations. Thus an effective assessment strategy must utilise a combination of methods, which accumulate data gathered from diagnostic techniques. Notwithstanding all of this it is an inescapable fact that, however sound the assessment strategy, the assessment of individuals in the ever-changing context of clinical practice requires the exercise of professional judgement.

## References

Bendall E (1975) *So You Passed, Nurse!* London: RCN

Bligh D (1975) *Teaching Students.* Exeter: UETS

Collingwood (1990) *Does it Work? An Investigation into the Use of Behavioural Objectives to Assess the Practical Elements of Nurse Training.* Unpublished MBA thesis, University of Edinburgh

Dreyfus S E & Dreyfus H L (1980) *A Five Stage Model of the Mental Activities Involved in Directed Skill Acquisition.* University of California: Air Force Office of Scientific Research

ENB (1991) *Professional Portfolio.* London: ENB

ENB (1993) *Regulations and Guidelines.* London: ENB

Falchicov N (1986) Product comparisons and process benefits of collaborative peer group and self assessments. *Assessment and Evaluation in Higher Education*, **11**(2): 146–166

Harrison R (1984) Accreditation, validation, evaluation and assessment. In Goodlad S, *Education for the Professions — Quis Custodiet.* Guildford: SRHE and NFER-Nelson

Hepworth S (1989) Professional judgement and nurse education. *Nurse Education Today*, **9**: 408–12

Hutchings M J (1981) A critique of Bendall's 'So you Passed, Nurse.' *Nurse Education Today*, **6**: 405–8

Kelly G (1955) *The Psychology of Personal Constructs.* New York: Norton

Kempa R (1986) *Assessment in Science.* Cambridge: Cambridge University Press

Lankshear A J (1990) Failure to fail. *Nursing Standard*, 4(20): 35–37

McHale M (1985) The importance of awareness. *Nursing Mirror*, **161**(18): 30–1

Mobley M, Emerson C, Goddard I, Goodwin S and Letch R (1986) *All About GCSE.* London: Heinemann Educational

Nicklin P J A (1984) *Description of Personal Construct Theory and its Potential Application by the Nurse Teacher.* Unpublished MEd assignment, University of Nottingham

Phillips T, Shostock J, Bedford H and Robinson J (1994) *Assessment of Competence in Nursing and Midwifery Education (Project 2000). Final Report of the ACE Project.* Sheffield: ENB

Pope M (1978) Monitoring and reflecting in teacher training. In Pope M L and Keen T R (1981) *Personal Construct Psychology.* New York: Academic Press

Ramsden P (1985) Student learning research: retrospect and prospect. *Higher Education Research and Development,* **4**(1): 51–69

Rowntree D (1987) *Assessing Students: How Shall We Know them?* London: Kogan Page

Schön D (1984) *Educating the Reflective Practitioner.* New York: Jossey Bass

Wood R (1987) *Measurement and Assessment in Education and Psychology.* London: The Falmer Press

# 7
# The Learning Environment

If learning were described as a permanent or relatively permanent change in behaviour resulting from experience, it follows that the characterstics of that experience are fundamental to the quality of learning. The notion that particular conditions or circumstances enhance or inhibit learning is not new. For over a decade there has been increasing scientific scrutiny of the milieu in which nurse training takes place. In particular the research of Orton (1981, 1993), Fretwell (1982), Ogier (1982, 1986) and Marriot (1991) illuminates the characteristics of clinical areas that provide a positive learning environment. In earlier studies the 'ward sister' role was confirmed as crucial in creating a climate conducive to learning. Orton's more recent (1993) work suggests that with the emergence of the ward manager role, it is the student's mentor who is the most significant role model. In this chapter the learning environment will be construed as those circumstances that directly or otherwise influence the teaching and learning of nursing. This deliberately loose definition, whilst embracing clinical experience, will permit discussion of other factors that influence the education of students.

## Creating the learning environment

In Chapter 11 issues relating to the validation of courses will be discussed in detail. It is necessary, however, at this juncture to consider the responsibilities of the course management team (CMT). The ENB (1993a) requires that a CMT be constituted to plan, develop, monitor and evaluate each course. Its membership, which includes practitioners, managers, students and teachers, has a fundamental responsibility for creating and nurturing an environment in which the curriculum will thrive. For this to be achieved the CMT must have not only a coherent philosophy and unambiguous terms of reference but also a common perception of what is meant by the term 'curriculum'. One popular definition of the curriculum suggests that it is 'all the opportunities planned for pupils by teachers' (Nicholls & Nicholls 1978). This all-embracing definition is seriously flawed: 'planned for pupils by teachers' casts students in the role of passive if not docile recipients and further implies that course planning is the exclusive responsibility of teachers. The discrepancy between what is taught and what is practised can only be widened if curriculum planning is perceived as a teacher-dominated, theoretical and academic activity. Although not a contemporary definition, Stenhouse's (1975) assertion that the 'curriculum is an attempt to communicate the essential features of an educational proposal in such a form that is open to critical scrutiny and capable of effective translation into practice' has, in the view of this author, weathered the test of transient fashionability and represents a pragmatic and robust view of what CMTs are in business for. Inevitably and reasonably members of a CMT will seek leadership on course design issues from educationalists. What is less reasonable is that the language, acronyms and regulations of education should bewilder and consequently impede practitioners, managers and students from making an effective contribution to course management. The legendary 'theory–practice' gap cuts both ways. Not only is it the responsibility of teachers to retain clinical credibility but also members of CMTs need to understand the educational principles underpinning the programmes they design and the professional and academic regulations governing the courses they manage. Too frequently non-teachers are appointed to CMTs without appropriate preparation for the role they are required to exercise. Appendix 1 is a glossary of terms and acronyms commonly encountered by CMTs.

Prior to the NHS reforms and the introduction of Project 2000 courses, clinical areas, particularly hospital wards, were highly dependent on student nurses as a source of labour. Subsequently with the shift of emphasis to care in the community, the substantial reduction in the number of hospital beds, changes in skills mix and the supernumerary status of students, placements are at a premium to meet the requirements of training rather than student labour to meet the demands of care. Since the implementation of Working Paper 10 (Department of Health 1989), there has been increasing pressure from some service providers to charge colleges for clinical placements that they regard as a cost to the service. Research conducted by a consortium of regional health authorities (NHS 1993) concludes: 'there is a net benefit to Trusts/Units providing clinical placements . . . benefits are largely long term quality effects while the costs tend to be more short-term and quantifiable'. Additionally, whereas previously the majority of clinical placements were within the NHS, experience is increasingly being gained in the independent and private sectors. What all this suggests is the need for greater clarity in describing the learning environment, the development of valid and reliable auditing procedures and the efficient and effective management of available clinical placements.

## Characteristics of the learning environment

The ENB's regulations (1993) require that 'an audit of practice placement areas must be conducted at least annually'. Audit has become singularly the most prominent technique for improving the quality of health and education sector services. In the context of clinical placements, it can be defined (adapted from NHSME 1991) as:

'Part of the cycle of quality assurance. It incorporates the systematic and critical analysis by Course Management Teams of clinical placements, in terms of the outcomes for students, and introduces appropriate changes to that analysis.'

Whilst auditing of placements should be undertaken at least annually it should also be conducted whenever the circumstances of a clinical placement change. Such circumstances would include a change of clinical manager, link teacher or clinical function. As new clinical services are developed, the CMT should participate with commissioning teams to assure that prospective placements meet the conditions of course validation. Occasionally a clinical placement may receive consistently low ratings from students or have a high absence and sickness rate. In these circumstances an audit may be undertaken for diagnostic purposes. An audit of clinical placements is typically undertaken by the ward manager, the link teacher, a student and a member of the CMT. The potential for educational audit to be an isolated and insular activity can be obviated by encouraging ward managers to audit each other's placements, through a system of 'peer review'. Placement audit should be assimilated within a hospital or unit's overall framework of nursing audit. This more open and comprehensive approach to audit enables the transmission of good practice, educational and clinical, to other placements and has the potential to minimise the 'theory–practice gap'. Similarly the audit of nursing and residential homes can be linked to the registration inspections conducted by health authorities and local authority social services.

In their *Guidelines for Educational Audit* (1993b) the ENB propose an extensive and comprehensive range of criteria for auditing practice placements. The ENB identify eight 'aspects of clinical learning that should be surveyed' and summarised in the annual report:

1 *Ethos of the placement:*
— general climate;
— channels of communication;
— approachability of staff;
— relationships between the college of nursing, midwifery/health studies;
— the placement, commitment to teaching and learning.

2 *Organisation of care:*
— individual approach to care;
— the organisation of workload so as to promote continuity, e.g. team nursing, primary nursing (midwifery, health visiting);
— involvement of student in multidisciplinary teamwork.

3 *Supervision and mentorship:*
— effectiveness of supervision and mentorship by first level nurses;
— contribution by academic staff;
— fulfilment of clinical contact hours;
— evaluation of compliance with statutory regulations in supervision and assessment of midwifery students.

4 *Teaching programme and assessment:*
— planned formal programme;
— opportunity for students to achieve continuous assessment of competences;
— the curriculum objectives and appropriate academic and professional level;

— compatibility of patient/client groups to support objectives at an appropriate academic and professional level.

5 *Research basis of care planning and delivery:*
— evidence of the application of research in teaching and implementation of care.

6 *Academic and professional qualifications of clinical staff.*

7 *Staff development programme.*

8 *Physical environment.*

Orton's (1993) research, published as *Charting the Way to Excellence — Indicators of Ward Learning Climate,* aimed to develop an audit tool to assess the quality of the learning climate. Orton and her colleagues identify six 'key issues' that characterise a good ward learning climate:

— *Orientation to the placement.* Students are welcomed to the ward and have a named mentor. Included within their orientation programme are written details of the ward's mission, policies and procedures.
— *Theory and practice.* There is a good relationship between the college and the clinical placement; what is learned in college is relevant to practice. Students are well supported and have adequate opportunity to participate in care that incorporates relevant research.
— *Supernumerary status.* Staff and students have common understanding of the student role. Students have opportunities to negotiate aspects of their placements and are not used merely as a 'pair of hands'.
— *Staff attitudes and behaviour.* Placement staff are approachable and supportive, and are well informed and positive about the course. Staffing levels are adequate, morale is high and the ratio of students to staff is appropriate. Students are encouraged to work with the ward team and ask questions, and are given adequate feedback on their performance.
— *The mentor.* The student has sustained exposure to a named mentor. The mentor is supportive, identifies learning opportunities for the student and is able to respond to differing learning styles of individual students.
— *Progressive assessment.* The requirements of placement assessment are agreed by the student and mentor, and progress is regularly reviewed. The student succeeds in achieving their agreed learning outcomes.

Orton's Ward Learning Climate Indicators are identified by the administration of a 55-item questionnaire to staff and students. An associated software package minimises the time-consuming process of scoring questionnaires and provides in graph form a summary of the learning climate (Fig. 7.1) and scores for items within each section (Fig. 7.2).

Ward Learning Climate Indicators for:

ward 8 sgh

Prepared on 02/11/93

**Summary**

A. Orientation to the placement

B. Theory and practice

C. Supernumerary status

D. Staff attitudes and behaviour

E. The mentor

F. Progressive assessment

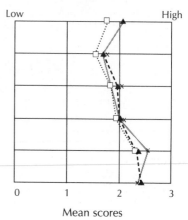

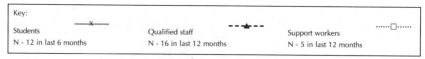

Fig. 7.1   Ward Learning Climate Indicators: summary chart

Ward Learning Climate Indicators for:

ward 8 sgh

Prepared on 02/11/93

**Orientation to the placement**

1  Staff welcome students on arrival

2  Students shown round ward

3  Students allocated mentor in first week

4  Students meet mentor in first week

5  Orientation programme on first day

6  Written communication before arrival

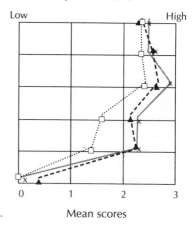

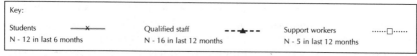

Fig. 7.2   Ward Learning Climate Indicators: section A chart

## Supervision and the learning environment

The clinical education of student nurses in the UK is substantially reliant on clinical nurses providing instruction and supervision whilst simultaneously managing and providing care in their clinical settings. Elsewhere, particularly in North America, placement supervision is the responsibility of instructors employed by schools of nursing. The debate on the appropriateness and effectiveness of the UK's model of student supervision is unlikely to abate in the foreseeable future. Whilst undoubtedly the clinical skills profile of nurse teachers must be improved — 'the teacher of the future should be first and foremost a practitioner' (RCN 1993); 'to enable teachers to maintain clinical practice, the equivalent of one day per week should be allocated to clinical activities' (ENB 1993a); 'The new framework (PREP) ensures teachers maintain clinical credibility' (UKCC 1994b) — the most significant and influential clinical role models will continue to be clinically-based staff. This is not to deny the considerable merit in the lecturer–practitioner role but, like its predecessor the 'joint appointment', it is possibly best perceived as an important but self-limiting strategy for enriching the learning climate. Such an assertion is consistent with Marriot's (1991) view that 'unless there is to be a drastic change in the role of nurse teacher or a considerable increase in their number, the role of mentor (clinical practitioner) is surely going to become more and more important'.

In the first edition of this book, the ward sister was described as 'the single most important person in creating a learning climate', although there was emerging evidence that students were becoming increasingly reliant on staff nurses for support, this being attributed to their role in recently introduced schemes of continuous assessment (Ogier 1986). Subsequently, with the emergence of the ward manager role, student and nurse education has sought to broaden its base for support and supervison. Jowett *et al* (1994) report a 'continuing downward delegation of managerial responsibilities, removing both ward managers and staff nurses further from direct patient (and student) contact'. Consequently whilst the ENB requires that students must have a first level nurse as a mentor, it concedes that other members of the nursing team contribute to the mentor relationship (ENB 1993a). A mentor is defined by the ENB as:

'An appropriately qualified and experienced first level nurse/midwife/health visitor who, by example and facilitation, guides, assists and supports the student in learning new skills, adopting new behaviour and acquiring new attitudes.'

Darling (1984) identifies what she considers to be the 'absolute requirements for a significant mentoring relationship', which are:

— *Attraction*: the student's admiration of the mentor and a desire to emulate him or her.
— *Action*: the mentor invests time and energy in teaching, guiding and helping the student.

— *Affect*: the mentor demonstrates respect, encouragement and support for the student.

Darling has developed and validated a 14-item Measuring Mentoring Potential (MMP) scale which could be used not only for assessing mentorship potential but also as a framework for designing mentorship programmes.

## Post-registration education and development

So far in this chapter the notion of a learning climate and concepts of supervision and mentorship have been discussed in the context of pre-registration nurse education. The dynamic nature of health care demand changes in systems of care delivery and advances in technology demand that nurses are constantly revisiting and revising their roles. The changes confronting nursing are logarithmic both in scope and pace. Whereas previously it was possibly justifiable to consider initial registration as an end in itself, it can now only be considered to be 'the end of the beginning' — the beginning of career-long professional development. This is accurately reflected in the UKCC's *Standards for Education and Practice* (UKCC 1993) which require:

— newly registered nurses to complete a period of about four months support under the guidance of a preceptor 'to ensure that practitioners do not take on too much responsibility too soon or inappropriately'. During this period of role transition practitioners remain accountable for their professional practice;
— practitioners to maintain and develop their professional knowledge and competence through a minimum of five study days every three years;
— nurses formally to notify their intention to practise every three years, providing details of qualification and area of practise when initially registered. These details are required when re-registering, re-entering practice after a break of five years or more or changing area of practice using a different registerable qualification. Midwives notify their intention to practise annually;
— completion of an approved return to practice programme and assessment of professional competence following a break in practice of five years or more;
— practitioners to maintain a personal professional profile to include experience, developments and achievements. The profile should be a dynamic means of recording career progress and contain details of continuing education, an assessment of educational and development needs and a plan to meet these needs.

The continuing professional development of the registered nurse is not exclusively the responsibility of the individual or their employer but of both. The individual nurse has the right to expect the provision of training opportunities, and the employer should require the nurse to maintain and develop the skills for which they are employed. This should not be a tacit agreement but a formal contractual obligation, exercised through a process of individual performance review (IPR). However the most commonly neglected feature of the IPR process is the construction of a meaningful personal development plan (PDP). The inclusion of the individual's professional profile (portfolio) in the IPR process will increase the precision with which training and development opportunities are prescribed. There is a tendency for appraisal to be viewed solely as a means of improving the appraisee's (nurse's) performance, rather than as an opportunity for focusing on the manager's development needs. Nicklin (1994) asserts that 'the IPR process should not focus exclusively on the achievement of individual objectives, but should be equally concerned with the quality and climate of leadership that facilitated or constrained individual employee performance'. Nicklin describes a system of 'employee appraisal of their managers' using a 20-item Likert-type scale (reproduced in Table 7.1).

Table 7.1  Quality of leadership questionnaire

Please rate your manager's leadership skills against the statements listed below. Attempt to provide a balanced appraisal, not being influenced by a specific or single positive or negative situation or event.

This questionnaire is anonymous and therefore entirely confidential. Your responses will be aggregated with those of your colleagues and the overall appraisal (mean x) fed back to your managers.

Circle the appropriate number on the scale 1—4.

| **My Manager:** | 4 Strongly agree | 3 Agree | 2 Disagree | 1 Strongly disagree |
|---|---|---|---|---|
| 1. listens effectively to others | 4 | 3 | 2 | 1 |
| 2. accurately reflects what others have said to check understanding | 4 | 3 | 2 | 1 |
| 3. asks open questions | 4 | 3 | 2 | 1 |
| 4. challenges what others have said in a constructive and non-threatening way | 4 | 3 | 2 | 1 |
| 5. consistently gives appropriate and unambiguous feedback to others | 4 | 3 | 2 | 1 |
| 6. acknowledges and praises what others do and say | 4 | 3 | 2 | 1 |
| 7. openly recognises and values the strengths and potential of others | 4 | 3 | 2 | 1 |

| | Strongly agree | Agree | Disagree | Strongly disagree |
|---|---|---|---|---|
| 8. is open to learning from subordinates | 4 | 3 | 2 | 1 |
| 9. makes clear and logical decisions | 4 | 3 | 2 | 1 |
| 10. has realistic expectations about my workload and time | 4<br>4 | 3<br>3 | 2<br>2 | 1<br>1 |
| 11. communicates plans and objectives clearly | 4 | 3 | 2 | 1 |
| 12. communicates up to date and relevant information | 4 | 3 | 2 | 1 |
| 13. has a clear sense of purpose and direction | 4 | 3 | 2 | 1 |
| 14. manages their own time effectively | 4 | 3 | 2 | 1 |
| 15. tackles issues 'head on' however difficult | 4 | 3 | 2 | 1 |
| 16. has a clear and consistent set of values | 4 | 3 | 2 | 1 |
| 17. is committed to our team | 4 | 3 | 2 | 1 |
| 18. is fair and impartial with team members | 4 | 3 | 2 | 1 |
| 19. delegates work appropriately | 4 | 3 | 2 | 1 |
| 20. makes themself available to team members | 4 | 3 | 2 | 1 |
| **Totals** | ____ | ____ | ____ | ____ |

Reproduced by permission of North Yorkshire College of Health Studies.

In the preceding sections the term 'supervision' has been applied to the mentorship in pre-registration education and implied in the description of the preceptorship relationship of the newly qualified practitioner. 'Clinical supervision' should not be confused with either. According to the Department of Health (1993a) clinical supervision is 'a term used to describe a formal process of professional support and learning which enables individual practitioners to develop knowledge and competence, assume responsibility for their own practice and enhance consumer protection and safety of care in complex clinical situations. It is central to the process of learning and to the expansion of the scope of practice and should be seen as a means of encouraging self assessment and analytical and reflective skills'. In *A Vision for the Future* (1993b) the Department of Health targets clinical supervison as a concept that 'should be further explored and developed'. Faugier & Butterworth

(1994), in a comprehensive review of the literature, define and describe models of clinical supervision and their applicability to nursing. They assert that 'nursing has been more likely to rely on the "exposure" to clients and the nursing environment rather than a formalised exposure to the expertise of more experienced colleagues'. In commending a 'continual learner' model of clinical supervision, they propose a 'composite model of clinical supervision which embraces the roles of mentor and preceptor and is continuous from pre registration training to post registration practice'. The authors conclude by recommending that statutory and professional organisations 'should urgently review the training implications of clinical supervision'.

Many contemporary organisations, including the NHS, regard themselves as 'learning organisations' and advocate career-long learning for their employees. The provision of apposite and comprehensive training and development does of course have revenue implications, particularly if staff have to be released from their duties. There is little point in making provision for training that nurses cannot attend due to a shortage of staff (Nicklin 1985):

'But I well recognise the ambivalence of the nurse manager. Releasing staff for training can overload slender staff resources; in contrast, not to release staff for training discourages nursing skills development. Faced with this dilemma, a manager may well ask if she is more likely to be criticised for being short of staff or short of skills — I suggest it would be the former.'

However training should not be considered as synonymous with absence from the workplace. Indeed a reasonable criticism of much training is that it is unreal, synthetic or an academic simulation. In recent years there has been a substantial increase in role-based, open and distance learning programmes, as employers and validators have acknowledged that a substantial amount of 'off the job' training is neither affordable nor credible. Such programmes include those offered by the Open University, Open College, Health Pickup and others. As a case history, the success of the Nursing Times Open Learning (NTOL) in providing accessible, affordable and credible conversion programmes for enrolled nurses is unparalleled. There has been not only a shift from 'college-based' to distance learning but also an increased emphasis on 'doing' rather than 'knowing'. Increasingly assessment of 'competence' through 'portfolio evidence' is displacing traditional examination methods. Indeed the cornerstone of the government's employment and training strategies, NVQs, are substantially based on the principle of workplace assessment of individual competence. The growth in distance learning and competence-based training possibly represents the most significant development in post-secondary education during the past 25 years. As such the profession should embrace, further develop and utilise these valuable techniques.

However a note of caution. These are adjuncts to existing methods and not a replacement for them. Distance learning has many benefits, including variable and flexible access, but should not be regarded as a cheap alternative to taught programmes. The preparation, publication and distribution of high quality distance learning materials is notoriously expensive. Nor should distance learning be used as a cynical means of shunting training from the workplace to the employee's home. Furthermore, individuals have preferred styles of learning; for some individuals, distance learning is less efficient than other methods. Similarly competence-based training and assessment, with its emphasis on employer-specified skills and workplace assessment of performance is intuitively a good idea. However Smithers (1993), in a comprehensive study, claims that whilst NVQs are proving popular, 'the great fear is they will turn out to benefit neither students themselves nor the country' and that they 'run the risk of merely occupying the time of a lot of people'. He concludes that NVQs are not raising vocational standards and asserts that 'our analysis suggests the reverse'.

## Adding up the past — professional and academic credit

The UKCC's *Standards for Post Registration Education* (1993) and the ENB's *Framework for Continuing Professional Education* (1991a) are complementary strategies for improving patient and client care by the provision of coherent, cost-effective, responsive and flexible education. Both the UKCC and the ENB emphasise the need to minimise 'repetitious learning', to gain academic credit in addition to professional recognition for courses undertaken, and the award of credit where learning can be demonstrated from experience (other than from a formal course of study). The vehicle for assembling evidence of learning and achievements is the individual's portfolio or profile, and the mechanisms for gaining credit are Accreditation of Prior Learning (APL), Accredition of Prior Experiential Learning (APEL) and Credit Accumulation and Transfer Schemes (CATS).

### The professional portfolio

For the purpose of this discussion the terms portfolio and profile are synonymous. Many employers have developed bespoke profile packs for their staff, and an increasing range is available commercially. The ENB (1991b), in introducing their 'professional portfolio', describe it as 'more than a straightforward recording device. It is also a way for you to develop skills of critical and reflective practice, to consider experiences in your professional and personal life and to evaluate the contribution those experiences make to your development and to improvements in client care'. A typical portfolio is described in Chapter 9.

In addition to meeting the requirements of effective registration, the portfolio will provide assessable evidence of learning, which may receive credit towards professional and academic awards.

### APL, APEL and CATS

These are seductively simple concepts. The principle of each is a concern for what has been learned, rather that where or how that learning has been achieved. The application of these principles however, is far less than simple:

— *Accreditation of prior learning (APL)*: a process by which individuals can claim and gain credit towards qualifications based on evidence from their past achievements, i.e. formal 'certificated' courses.
— *Accreditation of prior experiential learning* (APEL): evidence derived from non-formal forms of learning, often unplanned, through life experiences generally; this includes paid and unpaid employment and study that has not been 'formally' assessed.
— *Credit accumulation and transfer schemes* (CATS): systems by which APL and APEL are assessed and given credit towards an academic award. Credit points are awarded at a particular level depending on the complexity of the work or achievement. In England, Northern Ireland and Wales, the system is based on a notional three-year honours degree programme; in Scotland the system is based on a four-year honours degree. This credit system is summarised in Table 7.2.

Table 7.2  Credit system (adapted from UKCC 1993)

| Award | Credit points | Level of learning |
| --- | --- | --- |
| Certificate in higher education | 120 specific credits at level 1 | Level 1 — Knowledge of specific facts |
| Diploma in higher education | 120 specific credits at levels 1 and level 2 | Level 2 — Interpretation of facts |
| Ordinary degree | 360 specific credits: a minimum of 60 at level 3 and a maximum of 120 at level 1 | Level 3 — Application of knowledge |
| Honours degree | 360 specific credits: a minimum of 120 at level 3 and a maximum of 120 at level 1 | |
| Post-graduate diploma | 70 specific credits at level M (4) | Level M (4) — Analysis of knowledge |
| Masters degree | 120 specific credits at level M (4) | |

Instinctively, this all makes good sense, providing flexibility in mode, style and duration of learning, and transferability of studies, experience and credit from one situation or institution to another. In practice APL, APEL and CATS are complex and complicated procedures. Credit for learning cannot be claimed until it has been assessed and cannot be assessed until it has been identified. *Nursing Times* Professional Development (1994) identifies four stages in this process:

— Systematic reflection on experience.
— Identification of significant learning.

—  Identification of evidence to support claims.
—  Submission of portfolio or profile for formal assessment.

Most, if not all colleges and many employers now have specialist teachers or facilitators to assist staff to identify and prepare their portfolio evidence for assessment and credit rating. The decision to offer credit resides with the individual university or college. Whilst the principle of CAT schemes is universally understood and general guidance has been devised by the Council for National Academic Awards (superseded by the Open University Validation Unit), the UKCC acknowledges that 'institutions have their own methods of offering credit' and 'some institutions . . . are not open to negotiation'. But students seeking credit should not despair, as in health care there is an increasingly competitive market in higher education although some universities have been reticent in addressing CATS, others, particularly but not exclusively the new universities (the former polytechnics), have demonstrated a radical approach and devised progressive solutions to credit accumulation and transfer, without compromising academic standards.

Nursing, and therefore nurse education, competes with other disciplines and services within the health sector for scarce resources; in this respect demand will always exceed supply. Earlier individual performance review and personal development planning were commended as techniques for increasing the accuracy of training prescriptions. There is also a need to ensure that training represents value for money both for the organisation and the employee. The Quality Guide to Professional Development (Appendix 2) is intended to assist practitioners in selecting programmes that will meet their expectations. It is based on the 'QualEd' model described by Nicklin & Lankshear (1990).

## Stress and the learning environment

Almost 20 years ago, Birch (1975) speculated that anxiety was a significant influence on the withdrawal of students from nurse training, whilst Menzies (1961) had previously expressed her concern about the problem of stress in nursing. Subsequently the literature devoted to occupation-related stress among nurses has grown substantially. Hingley & Harris (1986) reported that 'the level of stress awareness in the profession is low. Rather than seeing stress as a solvable problem, the prevailing attitude seems to be either put up with the difficulties or get out'.

More recent evidence from the Institute of Manpower Studies (Seecombe & Buchanan 1993) and the Health Education Authority (1993) suggests that the situation has not been substantially improved. The HEA (1993) reports that, among other things, the culture of the NHS 'contradicts the promotion of reduced stress and contributes to unhealthiness at work'. Nurses confront suffering as few other people do; they are often expected to do the impossible in the way of providing comfort and care. Nursing is located within a large bureaucratic and rigid organisation that has lacked the security of an established and stable management structure for over a decade. Nursing transmits a culture of compliance; consequently the nurse may set unrealistic goals for herself, believing that she can accomplish an activity or feat in an unrealistic amount of time or against insurmountable odds. With respect to patient care, nurses expect themselves to be all things to all people and then chastise themselves when they fall short. The discrepancies between the values and behaviours learned in the school of nursing and those required in the work situation are well known, and this gulf between what is theorised and what is practised is a major source of stress for nurses. The student nurse is located in the midst of this perceptual conflict, attempting to make sense of her emerging nursing identity — no mean feat when one considers that many students are adolescent and seeking to establish their own individual identity.

In 1978 Shubin applied the term 'burn-out' to a syndrome promoted by job-related distress in nursing, the characteristics of burn-out being physical and emotional exhaustion, involving the development of negative self-concept, negative job attitudes and a loss of concern and feeling for clients. 'Stress' has a contemporary popularity amongst the ordinary public, educationalists and helping professions; it is possible to speculate that the phenomenon of burn-out is more apparent than real and simply promoted by the 'bandwagon' effect. Certainly, it is difficult to produce direct and objective evidence of burn-out. Burn-out is analogous to 'shell shock' or 'battle fatigue', and for many nurses to admit to burn-out would be synonymous with 'lacking moral fibre' and would offend the characteristic British solution to stress — the 'stiff upper lip'. Chambers-Clark (1980) describes a reluctance among nurses to legitimise their own right to health and well-being. This legitimisation may well conflict with meeting the emotional demands of patients and subordinates. Despite the difficulties in directly quantifying the incidence of occupationally-related stress, Nicklin (1987) and Hingley et al (1986) quite independently identified that workload, quality of relationships and conflicts and ambiguities of nursing roles were a significant source of stress. The majority of respondents in both studies considered nursing to be increasingly stressful. Preventing burn-out is infinitely preferable to treating it, especially as nurses are the health service's most costly resource and the cost of stress-related illness, absenteeism and inefficiency is a major drain on limited NHS resources.

Strategies for the prevention of stress can be classified as organisational or personal. While the organisation most certainly has a responsibility for diminishing stress, each nurse has an individual responsibility to prevent burn-out in herself. There is an inescapable paradox that stress to one nurse is satisfaction to another. Lazarus (1967) has demonstrated that a stressful situation cannot be defined by reference to objective criteria. Nicklin's (1984) research revealed the paucity of provision by health districts in preventing occupationally-related stress among nurses. In 1994 the Audit Commission reported, 'For too long the NHS has neglected its staff' and estimated that the cost of sickness absence among nurses exceeded £180 million a year, of which Rees (1994) estimates that 40% could be attributed to stress-related conditions, adding that student nurses were the health care group most vulnerable to the effects of work-related stress. This is a disappointing finding as, two years previously, the Department of Health had launched its 'Health at Work in the NHS' initiative, which included a commitment to 'promote positive mental health . . . and reduce sources of stress within organisations'. The NHS aspiration to promote healthy workplaces and be an exemplary and model employer is of course a long-term initiative, and its full benefits may not be evident for some time. The requirement of NHS units to include 'Health at Work' initiatives in their business plans will give additional leverage to the strategy.

Healthier workplace strategies that encourage employees to stop smoking, discourage the abuse of alcohol and advocate regular exercise and a 'healthy' diet are clearly welcomed, but they have a tendency to treat the overt symptoms of stress rather than addressing the underlying problem. Seyle (1956) suggests that individuals should develop a code of 'altruistic egoism' — a time-honoured procedure for managing stress — none of us can expect others to look after us more than after themselves! What is implied here is that individuals must accept responsibility for themselves. Birch's (1978) research revealed: 'The sample of students and pupils in this study emerges as a relatively anxiety-ridden group'. Birch concluded that a reform of the curriculum was required to provide students with the skills to meet patients' psychological needs. It is also apparent that whilst enabling students to meet the psychological needs of their patients, there is an urgent requirement that students should possess the skills to meet their own psychological needs. Clearly this assertion does not apply exclusively to students; as a contribution to curriculum building and the development of a 'healthy' learning environment, both pre- and post-registration courses should include self-management skills that will prevent occupationally-related stress. Techniques such as progressive relaxation, self-awareness, aerobics, assertion training and guided imagery have a legitimate place in health-based curricula. Continuing education is a prerequisite of a positive learning environment and should also be perceived as a method of preventing stress. Because a discrepancy between what is expected from self and others and the individual's current level of knowledge and competence can be stressful, continuing professional education can be perceived as not only a service-enhancing necessity but also a method of diminishing occupationally-related stress.

Of the range of potentially useful stress-reducing activities, support groups appear to have gained the greatest degree of acceptance in this country. Firth (1984) considers that personal support is just as important as adequate staffing. Mastach (1978) writes: 'Burnout rates are lower for those professions who actively express, analyse and share their personal feelings with colleagues. Not only do they get things off their chest but have an opportunity to receive constructive feedback from other people and to develop new perspectives of their relationships'. Hingley & Harris (1986) advise: 'We believe that all nurses should have access to a professional supervisor or mentor, someone within the workplace who can listen openly, challenge constructively and guide supportively'. In Chapter 8 the skills of listening and responding are considered in detail. Prophit (1981) reports that studies in longevity have cited two primary sociopsychological measures that are more predictive of long life than any other: work satisfaction and overall happiness. Yet work is a two-edged sword: It has the potential to enrich life but also the potential to create stress and suffering. The hypothetical relationship between arousal and performance is well known (Fig. 7.3). Arousal is essential for optimum performance, including learning; however as stress mounts, performance deteriorates.

The strength and success of curriculum delivery in nurse education is directly dependent on the environment in which teaching and learning takes place. Recent reforms of the health and education sectors, whilst posing problems, provide possibilities for enriching the learning environment. Eliminating the tensions between service delivery and the demands of the educational service remains a political conundrum. 'Students' however require the freedom to learn from competent role models in a stimulating and supportive environment where there is close proximity between nursing theory and nursing practice. In this context the title 'student' is not restricted to those who are about to enter the profession, but is expansive and applies to the 'professional student' — the nurse who exercises her professional accountability through career-long learning.

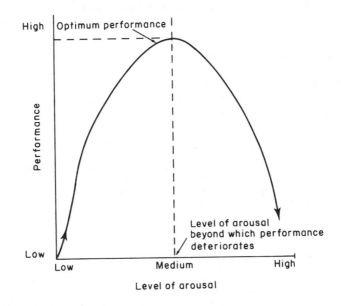

Fig 7.3    Yerkes Dodson Law — relationship between arousal and performance

# References

Audit Commission (1994) *Trusting in the Future*. London: HMSO

Birch J A (1975) *To Nurse or not To Nurse*. London: RCN

Birch J A (1978) *Anxiety in Nurse Education*. Unpublished PhD thesis, University of Newcastle upon Tyne

Chambers-Clark C (1980) Burnout — assessment and intervention. *Journal of Nursing Administration*. **9**: 43–49

Darling L A N (1984) What do nurses want in a mentor? *Journal of Administration* **Oct 14** (10): 42–4

Department of Health (1989) *Working for Patients*. Working Paper No. 10. London: HMSO

Department of Health (1991) *Framework of Audit for Nursing Services*. London: NHSME

Department of Health (1993a) *Clinical Supervision*. CNO (PL) 94(5). London:

Department of Health (1993b) *A Vision for the Future*. London: NHSME

ENB (1991a) *Framework for Continuing Professional Education*. London: ENB

ENB (1991b) *Professional Portfolio*. London: ENB

ENB (1993a) *Regulations and Guidelines for the Approval of Institutions and Courses*. London: ENB

ENB (1993b) *Guidelines for Educational Audit*. London: ENB

Faugier J & Butterworth T (1994) *Clinical Supervision*. Manchester: University of Manchester

Firth H (1984) Sources of good staff support. *Nursing Times*, **80** (18)

Fretwell J E (1982) *Ward Teaching and Learning*. London: RCN

Health Education Authority (1993) *Health at Work in the NHS*. London: HEA

Hingley P & Harris P (1986) Lowering the tension. *Nursing Times*, **83** (32): 52–3

Hingley P *et al* (1986) *Stress in Nurse Managers*. Project Paper 60: London: King's Fund Centre

Jowett S *et al* (1994) *Challenge and Change in Nurse Education*. Slough: NFER

Lazarus R (1967) *Cognitive and Personality Factors Underlying Threat and Coping in Psychological Stress*. East Norwalk, CT: Appleton-Century-Crofts

Marriot A (1991) The support, supervision and instruction of nurse learners in clinical areas. *Nurse Education Today*, **11**: 261–9

Maslach C (1978) *Job Burnout — How People Cope*. Public Welfare, Spring

Menzies, I P H (1961) *The Functioning of Social System as a Defence Against Anxiety*. London: Tavistock Publications

NHS (1993) *In the Balance*. Sheffield: Northern RHAs

NHSME (1991) *Framework of Audit for Nursing Services*. London: DoH

NHSME (1992) *Health at Work in the NHS — Action Pack*. London: HEA

Nicholls A & Nicholls H (1978) *Developing a Curriculum*. London: Allen & Unwin

Nicklin P J (1984) *Organisational Management of Nursing Related Stress in One NHS Region*. Unpublished M Ed assignment, University of Nottingham

Nicklin P J (1985) A case of mistaken responsibility. *Nursing Mirror*, **160** (19): 26–8

Nicklin P J (1987) Violence to the spirit. *Senior Nurse*, **6** (5): 10–12

Nicklin P J (1994) Internal Customers. *Nursing Times*, **90** (46): 46–48.

Nicklin P J & Lankshear A J (1990) Quality matters. *Nursing Times*, **86**: 31

*Nursing Times* (1994) Writing your portfolio. *Nursing Times*, **90** (14): 1–4

Ogier M E (1982) *An Ideal Ward Sister?* London: RCN

Ogier M E (1986) *An Ideal Ward Sister — seven years on*. *Nursing Times*, **82** (2): 54–7

Orton H D (1981) *Ward Learning Climate*. London: RCN

Orton H D (1993) *Charting the Way to Excellence*. Sheffield: Pavic Publications

Prophit P (1981) Burnout: the cost of involvement of being human in the helping professions. In Prophit P (ed) *Research: A Base for the Future*. Edinburgh: University of Edinburgh

RCN (1993) *Teaching in a Different World*. London: RCN

Rees D (1994) Report of Royal College of Physicians Conference. *Nursing Times*, **90**: 12

Seecombe I & Buchanan J (1993) *Absent Nurses: The Costs and Consequences.* Brighton: IMS

Seyle H (1956) *The Stress of Life.* Maidenhead: McGraw-Hill

Shubin S (1978) Burnout, the professional hazard in nursing. *Nursing*, **8** (7): 22–7

Smithers A (1993) *All Our Futures — Britain's Educational Revolution.* London: Channel 4 Television

Stenhouse L (1975) *An Introduction to Curriculum Research and Development.* London: Heinemann

UKCC (1993) *Standards for Post Registration Education.* RL 8 (93) London: UKCC

UKCC (1994a) *PREP 'Statement on Policy and Implementation'.* London: UKCC

UKCC (1994b) *The Future of Professional Practice.* 94/07. London: UKCC

# 8
# An Introduction to Counselling and Counselling Skills

The focus of this chapter is concerned with the skills of *helping others to understand themselves better and enabling them to be more effective in solving their problems.* As such it only aspires to be an introduction to the principles and practice of counselling. Although these skills will be discussed in the context of helping students, the principles are just as applicable to helping relationships with patients, colleagues and friends. Many student nurses are away from home for the first time and are in the process of resolving the normal emotional and social conflicts of adolescence and early adulthood. Others are 'mature students', making a career change or re-entering the labour market following a voluntary or enforced career break. They are subjected to the rigours of study and anxieties of examinations, in addition to experiencing at first hand the suffering and anguish of others. Unusual demands for pity, compassion and patience are made on students who may have inadequate experience or skills to cope with them, so it is hardly surprising that students encounter problem situations for which they require sensitive and skilled assistance. But who should assist? Helping and counselling are not the exclusive responsibility of those formally called and employed as counsellors; in this respect the Standing Conference for the Advancement of Counselling identifies three groups of helpers:

— people who are employed specifically as counsellors — referred to as 'professional counsellors';
— people for whom counselling is a legitimate and generally recognised, if subordinate, part of their role — referred to as 'counsellors';
— people who use counselling skills in the normal course of their working lives, possibly without recognising them as such — referred to do 'doing counselling' but not as being counsellors.

Briggs, Chairman of the Committee on Nursing (1972), expressed concern about the stresses of nursing and identified 'the creation of a comprehensive counselling service as an urgent top priority'. Almost a quarter of a century later, the stressors described by Briggs remain evident but the service he envisaged is conspicuous by its absence. In an earlier edition of its *Code of Professional Conduct* (1984), the UKCC required nurses to have regard for 'the workload and pressures' on colleagues and to take 'appropriate action'. The subsequent edition (UKCC 1992) is less explicit, merely requiring the nurse to 'report to an appropriate person . . . when the health and safety of colleagues is at risk'. However even if the service that Briggs envisaged existed today, students would still require the helping skills of their qualified colleagues. In the absence of such a service the basic skills of 'doing counselling' are even more necessary and fundamental to the trained nursing role.

The purpose of this chapter is therefore to enable trained nurses to reflect on their 'helping' or 'doing counselling' skills and, where appropriate, to encourage further skills practice to improve their counselling performance. The words of the previous sentence — 'to enable', 'to reflect', 'to encourage', 'to improve' — were carefully chosen, the reason being that whilst most people would not expect to be able to drive a car without training and practice, many individuals feel that interpersonal or 'people skills' should come naturally and therefore the suggestion of training in this area is a criticism of their personal qualities. Conversely training is considered to be some sort of remote and mystical process for a selected few. The evidence is that basic and effective helping skills can be substantially improved through training and practice and that these fundamental skills of helping can be developed by the average, healthy and caring individual. Of this situation Egan (1994) advises:

'although helping can and does work, there is plenty of evidence that ineffective helping also abounds. Helping is a powerful process that is all too easy to mismanage . . . helping is not neutral. It is for better or for worse.'

## Counselling theory and principles

Like other nursing activities, counselling is essentially a practical activity, and in the past there has possibly been a tendency to overload the prospective helper with psychological theory at the expense of skills training. However before proceeding to consider specific helping skills and training exercises, some guidelines and theoretical assumptions must be considered; indeed, 'there is nothing as practical as a good theory'.

The skills described in this chapter are biased towards a 'person-centred' and 'problem management' approach to counselling and as such are heavily influenced by the work of Carl Rogers and Gerard Egan. There are of course many theories of counselling and alternative approaches to helping. Frequently counsellors use techniques and principles derived from different theories in an eclectic fashion. A thorough review of these different perspectives is provided by Corey (1991).

*Basic assumptions*

The purpose of a 'client-centred' approach to counselling is to help the individual to help herself. Such an approach requires the 'client' to accept or 'own' her problem situation, to make a 'free choice' about solutions and to accept responsibility for the actions she takes to resolve her difficulties. The helper's responsibilities are to facilitate change by helping the client to explore her problems, to assist in identifying acceptable and workable solutions and to encourage the client to carry out whatever actions or solutions have been agreed. Helping, using this model, does not include:

—  *telling the client what to do*: 'If I were you I'd go and see the Director of Nursing Services and complain about . . .';
—  *analysing and explaining the individual's difficulties*: 'Ah! Well, you see your problem is that you've never cared for someone who is dying before, and the reason you're feeling guilty is because . . .';
—  *applying your solution to their problem*: 'I know exactly how you feel. When I failed my final examinations, what I did was . . .';
—  *being judgemental*: 'Well, that's a fine mess you've got yourself into. I can't imagine what you were thinking of. If you're expecting sympathy from me . . .'.

This last example illustrates one potentially major problem or obstacle in a helping relationship. In the health service there has been a tendency to use the term 'counsellng' to describe a procedure used in the disciplinary process; this activity would be more accurately labelled as a 'disciplinary interview'. Furthermore there is the problem of role conflict. A student may have personal difficulties that are reflected in unacceptable professional behaviour. The ward sister may simultaneously, as a manager, wish to discipline the student and also, as a helper, provide assistance. A student who has failed an assessment may seek help from his teacher, but, in addition to 'counselling', the teacher may be obliged to 'formally advise' the student that a subsequent academic failure will result in discontinuation of training. These quite different roles are not mutually exclusive, but they cannot be exercised simultaneously. Boundaries and terms of reference must be established so that both parties are quite clear about the objectives of their interaction. In many circumstances these dual roles can exist in parallel.

The notion of *confidentiality* is fundamental to the counselling relationship. Confidentiality is a complex issue, and it and other dilemmas of counselling cannot be resolved in one short chapter. Taylor (1983) makes two salutary observations:

'If you are genuine about making the client responsible for the content and disclosure in a session, then you must be prepared to take what comes.'

'What goes on in a session is not your property, it is that of your client, and you are not at liberty to use it in any way without his or her knowledge or consent. You are not on a fact-finding mission for another agency.'

For some there are no degrees of confidentiality — it is *absolute*; and on superficial examination this may seem not only reasonable but also the essence of a counselling relationship. However absolute confidentiality poses dilemmas for both helper and client. Having agreed to such a condition, if the client then discloses intent to endanger himself or others, or alternatively reveals evidence of exploitation of colleagues or clients, what then? Of this scenario Burnard (1992) suggests 'do not readily offer a confidential relationship if you feel that, in doing so, you may put yourself or your client at risk', the general principle being that information will only be passed on with the client's knowledge or consent. In this respect the UKCC's (1992) *Code of Professional Conduct* can be usefully paraphrased:

> 'Protect all confidential information and make disclosures only with consent, where required by the order of a court, or where you can justify disclosure in the wider public interest.'

### The helping relationship

A variety of characteristics are apparent in an effective helping relationship. Significant features of this helping climate are as follows:

— The relationship is empathic: the helper understands the experiences and feelings of the client and this understanding is conveyed by the helper.
— The client and the helper relate well to one other.
— The helper is sensitive to the client's difficulties and sticks closely to his problems.
— The client feels able to say exactly what he likes.
— The relationship is based upon mutual confidence and trust.

Rogers (1957) considers that three core conditions are necessary for the helper to be effective:

— *Genuineness* is about being authentic, being oneself and not employing façades. It requires openness, honesty and the use of appropriate self-disclosure. It means being spontaneous and not acting out some predetermined role or plan of action.
— *Unconditional positive regard* means demonstrating respect and non-judgemental acceptance of the client's dilemma. It means valuing the individual's unique nature and not applying conditions to acceptance. It is the ability to demonstrate to the client that he is worthwhile and has the capacity to overcome his current difficulties.
— *Empathy*. There is no 'objective reality': each of us perceives the world differently. Empathy means understanding clients' experiences and feelings from *their* frame of reference and entering into their 'reality'. It means conveying to clients that they are understood. Huxley (1963) notes: 'To see ourselves as others see us is a most salutary gift. Hardly less important is the capacity to see others as they see themselves.'

Of these Rogers considers empathy to be the central condition of the counselling relationship. Other observers collectively describe the three core conditions as 'basic empathy'. The evidence seems to suggest that these conditions are vital for a successful counselling relationship.

### Self-awareness

The major resource that a helper brings to the counselling relationship is himself; consequently, the more complete his understanding of himself, the greater his capacity for self-awareness and the more effective he will be as a counsellor. Helpers need to have a positive and accepting view of themselves. The individual who is self-deprecating is unlikely to promote self-acceptance in his clients. A healthy self-concept however is not based on an assumption or illusion but on self-examination. Individuals who acceptingly acknowledge the discrepancy between their 'ideal self' and 'real self', the person they would wish to be and the person they are, are more likely to have a positive view of the worth and dignity of others. Self-awareness also implies being aware of the limits of one's knowledge and ability; this may be reflected by the individual actively studying, undertaking further training or seeking the assistance of a more experienced colleague.

Of course self-awareness is not a quality that is specific to counselling; it is a prerequisite for all dimensions of helping. The view previously expressed in this book is that self-awareness is fundamental to the nursing role and therefore to nurse education. As such experientially-based self-awareness training should be placed to the fore in nursing curricula. The range of experiences for self-awareness training is becoming increasingly extensive: You and Me (Egan 1977) is a particularly useful training manual and includes many individual and group exercises, as in the following examples.

**Some questions about my interpersonal style (extract)**    (© 1977 Wadsworth Inc., Brooks/Cole Publishing Co, Pacific Grove, California, USA). Ask yourself the following questions:

How much of my day is spent relating to people?

Do I have many friends or very few?

Is my life too crowded with people?

Do I plan to get together with others, or do I leave getting together to chance — if it happens, it happens?

Do I choose to be with people who will do what I want to do?

Do I feel that I need my friends more than they need me, or is it the opposite?

Do I take others for granted?

Do others see me as self-centred? If so, how?

Am I my real self when I'm with others, or do I play games and act phoney at times?

Do I ever talk to others about the strengths and the weaknesses of our relationship?

Am I an active listener — that is, do I both listen carefully and then respond to what I've heard?

Do I enjoy it when others share with me whatever is important in their lives, including their secrets and their deepest feelings?

What people am I close to now?

Are there many different ways of being close to others? What are these ways?

Which ways do I prefer?

Is it easy for others to know what I'm feeling?

Do I try to control others by my emotions — for instance, by being moody? Do I manipulate others?

Does feeling left out and lonely play much part in my life?

Can other people scare me easily?

Do I ignore or reject others who might want to get closer to me?

Do I like to control others, to get them to do things my way? Do I let others control me? Do I give in to others much of the time?

Am I willing to compromise — that is, to work out with another person what would be best for both of us?

Do I feel responsible for what happens in my relationship with others, or do I just let things 'take their course'?

At school or at work, do I treat people as people or do I see them as just other workers or just other students?

Am I willing to allow others to be themselves?

In what ways am I too cautious or too careful in relating to others? What are my fears?

Do I share my values with others?

**Exercise**    Which questions did you find the most difficult to answer? Which questions would you be afraid to discuss in your training group?

**Exercise**    Using the set of questions as a guide, write a short, one-page description of your present interpersonal style. On the one hand write only what you would be willing to read or show to your fellow group members; on the other hand try to show a side of you that you think you do not usually let others see.

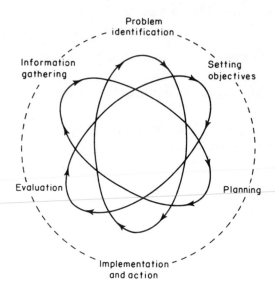

Fig 8.1    Problem-solving sequence

*A model of helping*

The model of helping proposed here is a 'problem management' or 'problem-solving' approach. In our everyday lives we use problem-solving sequences of the type illustrated in Fig. 8.1.

It is precisely the sequence applied to diagnosing and rectifying the problem with a car that will not start or to planning the annual summer holiday. It is also the approach advocated for the delivery of nursing care, where it is called the 'nursing process'. Frequently this sequence of events is described as a 'cycle', which implies uninterrupted passage from one stage to the next. For ease of expression and understanding this is very convenient, but it does conceal the dynamic relations of the various elements: quite frequently problem-solving plans have to be changed because 'new' information becomes available or an intended course of action is no longer possible, or alternatively what was previously considered to be a principal objective is eclipsed by another. Consequently each stage is in direct relationship with the others. In the next section of this chapter, the skills of helping will be discussed under the headings of a problem-solving sequence, but in reality the helper may well be using skills associated with different parts of the 'cycle' simultaneously.

*Summary*

In summarising this section on theory and principles of counselling and before proceeding to consider the practical skills required, it is worth reaffirming the purpose of the helping relationship.

In his three-stage model of helping, Egan (1994) describes the following helping framework:

— *Stage I: Reviewing the current scenario.* Clients' problem situations are explored and clarified. Clients cannot possibly manage problem situations unless they are understood. Identification of the problem is described as *the current scenario.*
— *Stage II: Developing the preferred scenario.* Goals based on an understanding of the problem situation are set — *the preferred scenario.*
— *Stage III: Getting there.* Action — ways of accomplishing goals are devised, implemented and evaluated. These are the means of moving the client from her *current scenario* to her *preferred scenario.*

## Counselling skills and practice

It is possibly self-evident that helping or counselling requires time, not necessarily a lot of time, but that time must be exclusively devoted to the client and be free of interruptions and distractions. Frequently ward offices are totally unsuited to this purpose. How much time is needed depends on a number of variables, not least how much time one can reasonably afford. A ward sister or a trained nurse is unlikely to be able to devote much more than 30 minutes on any single occasion to helping a student with a problem.

What is important here is that a boundary is set so that the client knows exactly how much time there is at her disposal. Additionally there must be clarity about the purpose of the meeting so that this cannot be misconstrued by the client. A 'person-centred' and 'problem-solving' model assumes that the client, aided by the helper, will assume responsibility for the management of her problem; consequently she needs to know how this can be achieved. The model does not belong to the helper and should not be concealed from the client. As a client group, students may have encountered 'models of helping' in their training, but even if they have not, they will easily assimilate the principles. All that is implied here is that if clients are to help themselves, it will certainly aid the situation if they know what is going on.

## Information gathering and problem identification

If the helper is to empathise with the client's problem situation, she must listen attentively and in turn confirm with the client that she has understood what is being said. Active listening conveyed by the helper and experienced by the client is a prerequisite of effective helping but is not as common as might be supposed. In theory a model of listening might be represented as in Fig. 8.2.

The process of listening to another person is often interfered with by our own thoughts, problems and feelings. When you are thinking about what you want to say, it is difficult to attend to what is being said.

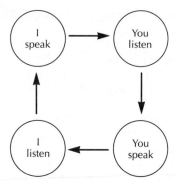

In reality the sequence is often:

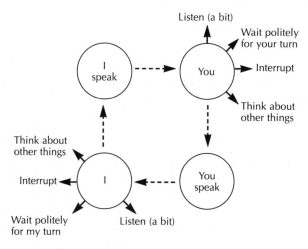

Fig 8.2    Model of listening

*Basic attention*

A fundamental requirement of the helper is to convey to the 'client' that she is being listened to. The experience of successful counsellors suggests that the following are useful.

— Maintain a comfortable distance, adopt a posture of relaxed alertness; face the client square on, leaning slightly forward; keep arms and legs unfolded.
— Maintain good eye contact, not a hard gaze but a soft, involved eye contact.
— Avoid extremes of movement such as fidgeting or sitting completely still.
— Avoid physical barriers such as a table or the arm or back of a chair.

A useful mnemonic for basic attention is *SOLER*:

**S**quare on, **O**pen posture, **L**ean forward, **E**ye contact, **R**elaxed

**Exercise**    In pairs, one partner is briefed to 'disclose' an issue that currently concerns her but is advised that this should not be too serious a problem. Separately the other partner is briefed initially to listen attentively to her partner's 'problem' but gradually to appear distracted and bored, to check her watch, occasionally look out of the window and so on. After five minutes the interaction is stopped and the partners discuss their experiences in turn.

### Minimum encouragement and silence

There is evidence that inexperienced helpers are eager to respond to their clients, to the extent that they may interrupt before the other person has finished what she wanted to say. However giving minimum encouragement by nodding, smiling, using sounds like 'Um-hmm' and 'Yeh' or comments such as 'I see', 'Do go on' and 'Yes', or simply repeating a word or two from the client's last phrase, has been demonstrated to increase substantially what the client has to say.

**Exercise**    In pairs, one partner is briefed to 'disclose' an issue of current concern to her but is advised that this should not be too serious a problem. Separately the other partner is briefed to use only minimal encouragement when listening. After five minutes the interaction is stopped and experiences are shared.

### Questioning

When gathering information and identifying problems, it is necessary for the helper to ask questions, particularly when the client finds it difficult to talk. However a series of unrelenting questions may be experienced by the client as an interrogation.

It is useful to distinguish between open and closed questions. Closed questions severely restrict the freedom to reply and tend to invite 'Yes' or 'No' or some factual information. This may be entirely appropriate at times, but a succession of closed questions is likely to accumulate information that is neither used nor understood. In contrast, open questions encourage the client to talk freely; such questions often begin with 'what', 'how' and 'could':

— 'What exactly do you mean by . . .?'
— 'What do you think would happen if . . .?'
— 'How do you feel when your patients . . .?'
— 'How has your attitude changed since . . .?'
— 'Could you tell me a little more about . . .?'

'Why?' questions are frequently used, but are possibly best avoided. 'Why?' questions require an explanation and, as many people are unaware of their precise reasons for their behaviour, are difficult if not impossible to answer.

**Exercise**    For a group of eight to 12 participants, prepare three piles of plain cards, with about 16 cards in each pile. On the cards of two piles write at random either 'Open' or 'Closed'. On the third pile write a series of general topics such as 'Horse riding', 'My summer holiday', 'Nurse education', 'Breakfast' and so on. Turn the three piles face down. One member of the group takes the top card from the topics pile and two others the top card from the other piles. The topic is read out and the members of the group are required to ask either an open or closed question about the topic as identified on the card. The process is repeated to involve all group members. The exercise concludes with members reflecting on the experience and discussing the ease and difficulty and the value and limitations of using open and closed questions.

**Exercise**    With a partner conduct a 'helping' interview, experiment with a variety of questioning techniques and record your questions and answers in the following way:

| Exact words used in the question | Outcomes in terms of length and quality of response | Is this an open or closed question? |
|---|---|---|
| | | |

*Reflection of content and feelings*

One of the indications of empathy is the ability to feed back to the client what has been said and the accompanying feelings that the client is expressing. Reflecting is a method of demonstrating that one understands without judging or evaluating what has been expressed. Reflections enable the client to see herself more clearly and assist the helper in checking that she really does understand. It is not always easy to sort out the feelings from the content that is being expressed; skilled helpers are able to do both simultaneously, although it may be more appropriate at times to focus on one rather than the other. From the point of view of training, it is useful to consider the skills of reflecting content and reflecting feelings separately.

*Reflecting content (paraphrasing)*

Paraphrasing is not merely repeating exactly what the client has said: it is the skill of putting the essential meaning of what has been said in other words. It might mean using a key word or phrase that seemed particularly important.

Client:    'Everything was going so well. I used to enjoy going out with my friends and really looked forward to work, but things are just falling apart. I've lost interest, I've no enthusiasm, I'm just low. I've been late on the ward twice recently and if I don't get down to some work I'm going to fail my exams, and that worries me a lot.'

Helper:    'So you've lost interest in things, it's affecting your work and you think you could fail your exams.'

When paraphrasing it is useful to be tentative which could mean prefacing the reflection with 'What you seem to be saying is that . . .' or concluding the reflection with 'Is that right?' This not only encourages the client to carry on but also conveys the concern that what is being said should be clearly and accurately understood. Individuals who are distressed and confused sometimes give rambling, even incoherent, accounts of their problems, and it is difficult for the helper to understand what is really being said. A simple admission such as 'I really do want to understand, but I'm not sure what you're really saying', apart from encouraging the client to restate the problem, is an indication of honesty and conveys genuineness and concern. Clarifying is a powerful way of focusing on the significant issues. It helps to move the conversation forward and assists the client to identify what she really wants to talk about. This is achieved through questioning, paraphrasing and reflecting feelings.

**Exercise**    In pairs, one partner talks about an everyday problem. The other repeats exactly what is said — 'parrots'. Roles are reversed. Partners then discuss their experiences.

**Exercise**    In a group of six to 10, the facilitator invites one member of the group to discuss a real but not-too-serious problem. The other participants actively listen. The facilitator randomly selects one of the group to 'paraphrase' what has been said. The accuracy of the reflection is checked out with the 'client'. The participant who was paraphrasing then describes a problem and so on.

### Reflecting feelings

Reflecting feelings is different from reflection of content, the emphasis being on the overt or underlying feelings in what the client is saying. This skill of reflecting focuses upon the emotions and feelings of the client; feelings inevitably play an important part in the problem that the client presents. This selective attention by the helper will encourage the other person to explore feelings rather than content. For example, using the previous illustration but this time focusing on feelings, the reflection might be:

Client:    'Everything was going so well . . . that worries me a lot.'

Helper:    'You're feeling down and when you think about your exams, that frightens you a lot.'

Again, it is useful to be tentative by prefacing the reflection with 'I sense you're feeling . . .' or 'I imagine that you feel . . .'. The client may have mixed or even conflicting feelings; reflecting these back helps the individual to clarify what are the important issues. Sometimes there is a difference between the feeling stated and those expressed non-verbally. It can be useful to confront the client with this discrepancy:

'You say when you think about your exams it worries you a lot, yet as you talk about it you seem perfectly at ease.'

**Exercise**   Feelings or emotions can be difficult to label and describe. In pairs, firstly 'brainstorm' and list as many feeling words as you can. You will probably have words like:

Happy, sad, ashamed, bored, insecure, afraid, angry, hurt, loving, confused, rejected, trusting, free, guilty, satisfied, distressed, amused

and many more.

Using your list incorporate each word into a sentence describing what was happening when you felt the emotion: 'I felt really happy when . . .'.

**Exercise**   Words are construed differently by different people — the same words can have different meanings.

In pairs, brainstorm a list of feeling words (as above). Alternatively using each word, describe how you feel when you have this emotion: 'When I'm sad, I feel really down, I don't feel too good about myself . . .'.

*Summarising*

Summarising brings all the facets of the conversation together. It is a natural way of bringing a session to a close or confirming in the minds of both participants at the start of a session what was said at a previous meeting. It is useful to encourage the client to summarise: 'So what do you think are the important things we've been talking about?' It also helps the client capture the essence of her difficulties and gives her a sense of movement towards solving whatever problem she has.

**Problem identification**

The first stage of the helping sequence has been concerned so far with developing a trusting relationship based on the helper's respect, genuineness and empathy with the client. The skills described have been concerned with understanding and appreciating the client's difficulties and enabling her to gain a greater understanding of her problem. The problem with problems is that they are frequently expressed in vague terms, but if specific action is to be taken the problem has to be stated specifically:

Vague:      'I've had enough.'
Specific:   'I find nursing elderly people very stressful.'

Furthermore problems rarely have clear and simple solutions; if they had they would not be problems.

Problem: 'I started smoking six months into my training and can't give it up.'
Solution: 'Stop smoking!'

Another problem with problems is that there are frequently secondary rewards in the behaviour that is considered to be a problem. The client needs to be helped to understand what these rewards are if she is to deal with her difficulties more effectively. At this stage the client may evade the problem or simply blame her dilemma on other people.

'Sister's always finding fault, it really screws me up, that's what makes me smoke.'

An appropriate and sensitive reflection will help the client to challenge the way she is managing her situation.

'So, it's Sister who makes you smoke?'

*Challenging* is a powerful technique for moving clients forward; however if used to 'shock', or if used insensitively and inappropriately, it will have negative and regressive consequences instead of helping the client.
     Finally the client has to 'own' the problem — it is hers and it is her responsibility. Of course identifying and owning a problem does not actually change a thing. Not infrequently counselling stops there, occasionally because the client feels the consequences of change are worse than the current situation (scenario) but more frequently because the helper, having talked through the problem, leaves the client to 'get on with it'. Understanding the problem is essential, but on occasion far too much time can be spent wandering around and around in Stage I, repeatedly examining, refining and defining the problem (Egan 1986):

'Assessment for the sake of Assessment, Exploration for the sake of Exploration, and Insight for the sake of Insight are all useless; they are successful to the degree that they enable the client to construct a more desirable scenario in terms of realistic goals or objectives.'

Many students who seek or require assistance have thought deeply about their difficulties, have mentally rehearsed what they want to say and are intelligent and articulate. Consequently problem identification might be achieved relatively quickly. The issue now is:

'If it weren't this way — how would it be?'

## Setting objectives and planning

Once the client understands her problem situation, she may need assistance in identifying realistic objectives. Such objectives should reveal an awareness of the following:

— Clients can be overwhelmed by the magnitude of the task ahead. Objectives should be broken down into units that are workable and that clients feel they can manage.
— The individual needs to know clearly what the target is and whether or not it has been achieved. Objectives should be unambiguous and stated in a behaviourally descriptive way so that achievement is measurable.
— The client owns the problem; she must also own the objective, and therefore it must be acceptable to her if she is committed to attaining it.

Objectives should always be elicited from the client and not given by the helper. The counsellor can encourage the individual to brainstorm alternative objectives, although these may well be limited and painful choices will have to be made. The helper can assist here by encouraging the client to consider the consequences of her actions. Expedient short-term solutions may ultimately pose long-term complications and difficulties. Once all the potential objectives have been examined, the client needs to make a decision based on her own priorities. During this step the helper's role is to encourage the client to make a choice and, once this is made, to help the client commit herself to it. One useful strategy for reinforcing the client's commitment is to examine those factors that will help her to reach her objective and those that might hinder her progress. Again the client is encouraged to brainstorm, on this occasion all those factors, direct and indirect, that will help to achieve the objective and then the factors that hinder or restrain progress. It is useful if the client writes these down, not only so that factors are not forgotten but also because seeing the problem, the objective and the factors that will help or hinder on paper can reassure the client that progress is being made (Fig 8.3).

Of course some of these factors are more important or more powerful than others, and it might be useful for the client to underline those factors that will most strongly influence movement towards or away from the objective, as these will certainly influence her plan of action. The plan of action is concerned with *maximising* those factors that will help progress to the objectives and *minimising* or neutralising factors that will hinder. Whilst objectives describe the desired outcome, the plan identifies the steps to be taken to achieve it. Using the previous example the plan agreed by the client might be as shown in Fig. 8.4.

As the plan has been discussed from the point of helping and hindering factors, it could be a list of 'dos' and 'don'ts'. It is useful if a plan is stated in positive action terms — doing.

## [Problem: I haven't prepared for my examinations]

| HELPING FACTORS | HINDERING FACTORS |
|---|---|
| 1  I want to be a registered nurse | 1  I get bored easily |
| 2  Explain problem to boyfriend | 2  I like going out |
| 3  Get someone to help me with a study plan | 3  I'm tired when I finish on the ward |
| 4  Find some quiet place to work | 4  My boyfriend complains if we don't go out |
| 5  Making a contract with myself to study each day | 5  I don't know where to start |
| 6  Ask people to be quiet | 6  My flatmates are noisy |
| 7  Join a tutorial group | 7  My friends will think I'm a 'swot' |
| 8  Go out less often | 8  Nobody else seems to bother studying |
| 9  Get my boyfriend to help me study | 9  I'm not sure it's worth all the effort |
| 10  Keep a progress chart | |
| 11  It will improve my job prospects | |

Objective:
Within one week to have developed and commenced a scheme of study

Fig. 8.3    Helping and hindering factors

| ACTION | ACHIEVEMENT DATE |
|---|---|
| 1  With personal teacher, undertake appraisal of areas of strength and weakness | Day 2 |
| 2  Prepare study scheme based on above appraisal: two hours each day | Day 3 |
| 3  Go out three times a week and relax —- a reward for keeping up with (2) above | Day 7 or sooner |
| 4  Discuss with boyfriend — ask for help, generally and with revision — be assertive | Day 4 |
| 5  Ask neighbours to respect my right to reasonable peace and quiet | Day 5 |
| 6  Keep a visual progress chart so I know what I've achieved | Now |

Fig. 8.4    Action plan

It is not necessary for the client to express formally her plan as illustrated above, although when this is done it has a contractual quality — the client contracting with herself to take specific actions by a predetermined date, the helper acting as a 'witness'. This reinforces the commitment to achieve the specific goals in an agreed time.

**Exercise**    In pairs, using the following 'problems':

I am overweight.
I smoke.
I can't seem to relax.
I don't have enough time for my family.
I am always in debt.
. . . and others you might think of.

Brainstorm as many objectives as you can for each problem — let your imagination run free, be creative.

## Implementation and evaluation

The client now has an understanding of her problem, has declared objectives for change and has devised a plan that will achieve the objectives. Although much progress has been made by this stage, the client's difficulties will remain unresolved unless the plan is implemented. The role of the helper at this stage is to encourage and support the client to take the planned course of action, which often means applying new or unused behaviours; permanent or relative changes in behaviour are called learning. Consequently the helper can at this stage usefully apply learning principles — these were discussed in Chapter 3. However it is useful to reiterate the motivating power of 'knowledge of results' and 'positive reinforcement'. At times it is not easy, from the client's perspective, to see exactly what progress is being made. The helper may assist by providing evidence of achievement: reward or 'positive reinforcement' is fundamental to behavioural change. The client needs to build rewards for success into her plan, and the helper, through approval and encouragement, can provide reinforcement and assist in shaping the desired behaviour.

### Role-modelling

A helper cannot be all things to all men (and women). However through her interaction with her client, she can demonstrate (model) useful interpersonal behaviour. Earlier in this chapter it was suggested that helpers should be 'self-aware', one component of which is being assertive in relationships. Assertiveness needs to be distinguished from other styles of behaviour:

— *Aggressive*: forcing people, attacking, intimidating, blaming, giving orders, dominating, violating the rights of others.
— *Manipulative*: deceiving others, insincerity, being two-faced, using people, making others feel guilty.

— *Submissiveness*: putting yourself down, not saying what you want, giving in, giving up responsibility, violating your own rights.
— *Assertive*: being honest in relationships, having respect for self and others, making own decisions, accepting praise and criticism, neither violating one's own or another's rights.

The helper needs to be assertive in implementing her plans, so do clients. There is evidence that student nurses are encouraged to be submissive (Briggs 1986). Indeed, some of their difficulties may be directly associated with being insufficiently assertive, allowing themselves to be dominated and manipulated. The client may vicariously learn useful styles of assertion through the behaviour of her helper.

## Role rehearsal

It is helpful if the plan is viewed optimistically but realistically as the helper can encourage the client to anticipate snags and obstacles. It can be useful if the helper and the student explore these, possibly by role-playing the potential difficulties. For example using the earlier illustration, the student may rehearse responding to a phone call when her boyfriend attempts to coerce or manipulate her into abandoning her planned evening of study so that they can go out for a drink.

Finally the effectiveness of the planned actions needs to be evaluated; the helper, with the client, can identify intended and unintended outcomes. If the client has failed to achieve her goal, it may be because circumstances have changed and the plan would require amendment to take account of this. Alternatively action might not have been taken because the plan was unrealistic or because the client has avoided taking the agreed action. In this situation the helper, whilst being supportive and acknowledging the achievements that have been made, can sensitively challenge the client. Considering evaluation, Connor *et al* (1984) suggest that the skills in this situation are being able to summarise and maybe challenge in a tentative way. Positive reinforcement should always be given at this stage, even in the face of apparent failure; for example the client should be rewarded for coming back to keep her appointment! New shaping strategies may then be worked out to help the client achieve the new objective and regain momentum.

Helpers can experience some difficulty in terminating a session or the helping relationship itself. In some respects this is even more difficult for the ward sister 'doing counselling' than the 'professional counsellor', not because of different skills levels but because of her day-to-day working contact with the client. The problem here is essentially one of managing boundaries; this includes boundaries of space (where we meet), boundaries of time (for how long we meet) and boundaries of role (why we meet). Some initial suggestions have already been made about the first two boundaries. The relationship is sometimes terminated because the client does not keep her appointment. However impolite or insensitive this may seem, it is the individual's right to terminate the helping relationship. If it is evident at the first meeting that it will be helpful to meet on future occasions, a boundary can be set: 'Shall we meet for half an hour once a week for the next three weeks?' This usefully identifies a potential point for termination. The boundary can always be adjusted in the light of experience, although it is unlikely that a trained nurse would be able to enter into a long-term 'counselling relationship' with a student. However relatively short-lived helping relationships are difficult to terminate; but if they are not terminated, there is the potential to create role confusion for future work encounters between the trained nurse and the student. Endings are never entirely satisfactory and 'goodbyes' are very difficult, but when the problem-solving work is done it needs to be acknowledged. At the final meeting it is useful to discuss openly feelings about termination before formally parting and reverting to the respective working roles.

**Exercise**    In threes (trios). This training exercise can be used to practise one specific skill or a series of skills. The three participants adopt the role of (1) client, (2) helper and (3) observer. These roles require:

— the *'client'* to present, preferably, a 'real' problem that is not too serious, which she feels confident in disclosing to the trio;
— the *'helper'* to practise and demonstrate a skill such as 'reflecting feelings', using the client's material;
— the *'observer'* unobtrusively and actively to observe the interaction between the helper and the client.

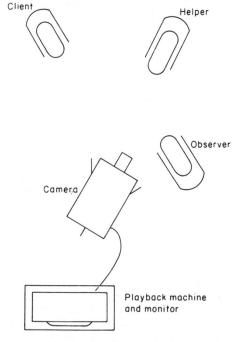

Fig. 8.5    Layout for videotaping an exercise

The client–helper interaction lasts 15 minutes and is then stopped by the observer, who gives feedback to the helper. Feedback should be based on what happened and on specific observed behaviours and should encourage self-assessment by the helper; the observer's role is not to give advice or to suggest how the interaction should have been managed. Feedback should last for five minutes. The participants then change roles. This exercise can also be augmented by the use of video so that participants can collectively or individually review the interactions (see Fig 8.5).

## Skills training

In this chapter an attempt has been made not so much to discuss the theory of counselling but to describe the practical skills that can be employed in helping. Some suggestions for skills development exercises have also been made. Like other skills 'counselling' can be improved by practice and by helpful feedback on performance. Counselling programmes ranging from introductory courses to masters level studies have proliferated in recent years. Most follow this sequence:

1   *Theories and principles* — through reading, lectures and seminars.
2   *Observation* — observing skilled practice either 'live' or using video. This provides behavioural clarity to the theoretical concepts learned above.
3   *Skills practice* — trainees practise skills under competent supervision (in trios for example) and receive helpful feedback, enabling them to shape and refine their skills.
4   *Maintenance* and development — continuing to develop understanding and skills, through lectures, seminars, their own practice and the shared experience of colleagues.

In 'taxonomic' terms the following progression is evident:

1   *Exposure* — the individual is introduced to the concepts of counselling as a 'student' or as a 'client'.
2   *Participation* — the individual commits herself to developing her own skills, there being a conscious effort to replicate the abilities of a 'role model'.
3   *Identification* — the individual commences training and commits time, intellect, emotion (and finance) to skills development.
4   *Internalisation* — the individual is active and self-directive; 'counselling' values characterise the individual's life style and behaviour.
5   *Dissemination* — the individual commends these skills to others, continues to develop her own skills and actively participates in the training of others.

For many nurses 'counselling' may be an occasional activity, for others a more frequent undertaking. In Chapter 7 the issue of 'supervision' was discussed, and the same principles are applicable to counselling. The paradox of much professional practice is that the 'novice' is trained in public and the 'expert' practices in private — behind screens or the classroom or office door. Russell (1993) proposes a client-centred model of supervision and asserts that 'supervision is an integral necessity for any worker in the caring professions, to ensure the best quality service for clients and the best quality development opportunities for workers'. In short, 'counsellors' require and should seek structured opportunities to reflect with peers or more experienced colleagues on their counselling practice.

In concluding this chapter on counselling skills, the reader is invited to assess his or her own skills using the rating scale shown in Fig. 8.6.

### SELF-ASSESSMENT

This rating scale is designed to assist you identify the 'micro' skills of the counselling process with which you feel confident and those which may require further skills development.

|  | Strongly agree | Strongly disagree |
|---|---|---|
| 1  I am the type of person that people approach when in 'trouble'. | I..........I..........I..........I..........I | |
| 2  When 'counselling' I always ensure 'boundaries' of time and space. | I..........I..........I..........I..........I | |
| 3  I listen actively to what people say. | I..........I..........I..........I..........I | |
| 4  My 'non-verbal' style conveys active attention and concern to the 'client'. | I..........I..........I..........I..........I | |
| 5  I am able accurately to reflect what the client has said without changing the essential meaning. | I..........I..........I..........I..........I | |
| 6  I can construct open questions that move the conversation forward. | I..........I..........I..........I..........I | |
| 7  I can use silence effectively in the helping process. | I..........I..........I..........I..........I | |
| 8  I am able to detect and label clients' feelings accurately. | I..........I..........I..........I..........I | |
| 9  Despite my own values I am non-judgemental of 'clients'' views and behaviours. | I..........I..........I..........I..........I | |
| 10  I can helpfully summarise what the 'client' has said. | I..........I..........I..........I..........I | |
| 11  I am prepared to disclose things about myself if necessary. | I..........I..........I..........I..........I | |
| 12  I am able to disassociate my role of 'manager' from that of helper. | I..........I..........I..........I..........I | |
| 13  I am able to end a counselling session/the helping contract in a positive way. | I..........I..........I..........I..........I | |

Fig. 8.6 Counselling skills — a rating scale

# References

Briggs K (1986) Speak your mind. *Nursing Times,* **82** (26)

Briggs A (1972) *Report of the Committee on Nursing* (Briggs Report). London: HMSO

Burnard P (1992) *Counselling — A Guide to Practice in Nursing.* Oxford: Butterworth-Heinemann

Connor M *et al* (1984) *Listening and Responding: Communications Skills in Nursing Care.* St John: The College of Ripon and York

Corey G (1991) *Theory and Practice of Counselling and Psychotherapy.* Pacific Grove, California: Brooks-Cole

Egan G (1977) *You and Me.* Monterey: Brooks-Cole

Egan G (1994) *The Skilled Helper,* 5th edn. Pacific Grove, California: Brooks-Cole

Huxley A (1963) *The Doors of Perception.* New York: Harper and Row

Rogers C R (1957) The necessary and sufficient conditions of therapeutic personality change. *Journal of Consulting Psychology,* **21**

Russell J (1993) *Out of Bounds.* London: Sage

Taylor B (1983) *Working with Others: Aspects of Helping and Counselling.* York: Oasis Publications

UKCC (1992) *Code of Professional Conduct,* 3rd edn. London: UKCC

# 9
# Recording and Reporting

There is a variety of reasons why those engaged in the enterprise of nurse education should keep records. Chapters 5 and 6 on assessment have dealt with the documentation and recording of educational outcomes. Similarly the chapters on quality (2), the learning environment (7) and evaluation (10) provide examples of record-keeping in specific circumstances. Recording information, impressions and incidents also facilitates *reflection on practices*. Reflective practice as a principle of learning was described in Chapter 3, and much that follows should be viewed in that context.

## Record-keeping and the student

Students keep records for various purposes to augment the learning process. The most obvious and most common is as an *aide mémoire*. Experience and information are not necessarily encountered as predicted by course planners; consequently the habit of maintaining a 'diary' on paper or by electronic means ensures accurate retrieval of information when required at some stage later in a programme of study. A second and significant use of record-keeping may be illustrated by the student who is interested in being able to compare such things as performance knowledge or feelings as she progresses through a course or course unit. It may be that she has been present when a patient has died. Knowing that this is not an uncommon occurrence in some areas of care provision, the student may wish to keep a record of her thoughts and feelings that surrounded the occasion. Subsequently when a similar situation is experienced, it may be helpful to the student again to record the associated emotions and compare them with earlier experiences.

Many students may keep copious records of their daily activities in both practical settings and study periods. This will prove to be beneficial, but only if the detail recorded is significant and related to the learning objectives being achieved. Recording irrelevant data is not only a waste of time but can disguise or detract from the important facts that should be understood and retained. The role of the nurse who is supervising the student must be not only to give sound guidance on what the student should record for learning purposes but also to check the material recorded at frequent intervals during the unit of experience. Another important aspect of written records is that of *confidentiality*. The qualified nurse must at all times impress upon the student the importance of using recorded information about patients only for her own educational purposes, not to divulge any part of such information and indeed not to leave the records unattended where they may be either lost or seen by unauthorised people.

A further reason why the student may wish, or be asked, to keep records is if she is to contribute to either the evaluation of that part of the course or a review of the ward or department as an effective care environment.

## Record-keeping and the supervisor

Supervisors of students, whether they be ward sisters, community nurses, staff nurses or midwives, will no doubt keep records of individual students to whom they act as mentors. Additionally the supervisor may keep records of the experiences encountered by the students so that each can be judged as to its value in providing sound learning opportunities and reinforcing good practice.

The relevance of maintaining continuous records of a student's performance becomes obvious when, at the end of an allocation period, the supervisor has to prepare a report about the student or award a score or grade to aspects of performance. In the absence of regular records of student progression, it is all too easy to recall either the instances of weak knowledge, mistakes in carrying out a nursing procedure or a faulty attitude, and pay undue attention to them, when in reality they were the exception rather than the rule. That is not to ignore their significance: the supervisor must draw them to the student's attention. However they can be seen out of overall context and detract from the strengths displayed by the student. The converse is equally important, and the isolated moment of brilliance must not be allowed to overshadow an otherwise unsafe and unsatisfactory performance.

Accurate and well-maintained records will be invaluable when arriving at an end-of-unit appraisal. Records on their own or taken out of context can be misleading or meaningless, but used in conjunction with other information they may reveal strengths and weaknesses or assist in problem identification. If the supervisor maintains a record of the student's pattern of timekeeping, what might this reveal over a period of, say, two to three months? Occasional late arrivals for early duties may be due to no more than late nights and an inability to rise early, but when linked with lateness for afternoon duties, 'pinching' the extra 10 minutes at meal breaks, eagerness to go off duty early and the occasional day's 'ringing in sick' with vague symptoms, this may reveal a more serious problem. It is very rare in this type of behaviour pattern to see a high level of performance and learning achievement within the student's progress. Mediocre standards of care, apathy towards learning and unacceptable attitudes to peers and supervisors are more readily observed.

Having put all these symptoms together by using accurate records, it remains for the supervisor, in conjunction with the personal teacher, to make a diagnosis and agree an appropriate action. Too frequently a student's sustained unsatisfactory performance is well-known but little understood due to the absence of accurate records, the worst possible scenario being Lankshear's (1990) 'failure to fail' described in Chapter 5.

## Record-keeping and the nurse teacher

Most nurse teachers are involved in a system that offers every student a personal tutor facility, and have responsibility for 20 or more students at any one time. It is likely that the nurse teacher will act as personal tutor to each student for the whole length of the course. Comprehensive record-keeping can help the teacher to maintain an accurate profile on each student, with a better chance of anticipating problems and offering appropriate solutions if the profile begins to reveal a deceleration in academic or clinical performance. Approaching the end of the course, the student will probably be applying for a staff nurse post, and it is likely to be the personal tutor, in conjunction with the course director, who will be asked to supply a reference in support of the student's application. Whilst formal records of the student's progress will be referred to, it is often the information of a less formal type available from the personal tutor that is of equal significance. The tutor who keeps records of this type can often provide information about a student that may be of use in a wide range of circumstances other than providing references for future appointments. Selection for special awards and membership of committees, working groups and curriculum teams are realistic examples of how recorded information about students can be put to practical use.

Reference has already been made to the other role of the nurse teacher, that of course director, where the teacher acts as the visible head of the course and ensures its smooth running by coordinating all of its component parts. Record-keeping, other than the statutory and formal records of the course and its students, may again be of real value. A weekly or even daily jotting down of any significant occurrences, good experiences, bad moments, disasters and the like can assist the course tutor with periodic review and evaluation of course units by augmenting or assisting in the completion of formal evaluation documentation. At a less formal level, the course teacher can refer to his records when selecting 'horses for courses' — which student to participate in which particular learning environment. Matching personalities, optimising learning opportunities, creating maximum cooperation between students and facilitating good group dynamics, all are made that much easier through the use of good information. Record-keeping need not be the sole property of the allocations officers, clerical staff or managers: the nurse teacher can also use it to great effect.

## Methods of recording information

### Professional portfolio

The UKCC's standards for education and practice (1994) require that practitioners maintain a professional portfolio. A portfolio is a dynamic means of recording career progress and contains details of continuing education, an assessment of educational and developmental needs and a year by which to meet these needs. It is also a means of developing the skills of critical and reflective practice. A typical portfolio will contain details of:

— *academic achievements*: secondary education, further and higher education;
— *professional qualifications*: registerable, recordable, other;
— *the professional employment record*: appointments, achievements;
— *continuing education and development*: study days, seminars, other learning experiences;
— *reflective practice*: a record and analysis of 'critical incidents';
— *a personal development plan*: objectives, planned experiences.

*Curriculum vitae*

A curriculum vitae (CV) can be best described as a selective synopsis of a professional portfolio and may be prepared for a number of reasons, most commonly as part of an application for a job or a place on a course. More popular than the formalised application form, the CV provides the applicant with a greater degree of flexibility and a better opportunity to present relevant information. It follows from this that the content of a CV will most likely change on each occasion that one is required.

A CV will normally contain the following information (adapted from Kenworthy 1993):

— Personal details

Name and home address
Telephone number
Date of birth
Whether a holder of a current driving licence

— General education

Formal qualifications attained: secondary, further, higher
Name of qualification
Place of study
Subject      Grade      Year
Highlight any significant achievement or award

— Professional education

Qualifications gained
Registerable      Recordable      Other
Name of qualification
Place of study
Year      PIN
Highlight any special achievements as a result of studies

— Previous employment

Years      Title and place of post      Employer
Briefly describe each post and key responsibilities

|   | | Highlight any special achievements or experiences in relation to previous posts |
|---|---|---|
| — | Relevant professional development activities | Be selective in describing those continuing professional education activities that you feel are relevant to the purpose of the CV<br>Highlight any significant achievements or experiences |
| — | Current post | Date commenced    Title and place of post<br>Employer<br>Work address and telephone number<br>Give brief account of your role and responsibilities, particularly if they are relevant to the purpose of preparing the CV |
| — | Other relevant details | Briefly describe any general or specific interests, pastimes, memberships, etc. |
| — | Key personal and professional features relevant to the reason for the CV | If the CV is being prepared as an application for a post or place on a course, it is appropriate to offer an account of one's characteristics and qualities that seem to present the best possible case for selection |
| — | Referees | Unless the type of referee required is specified, usually the current manager/employer, a person who can most convincingly promote your professional abilities and qualities should be sought |

There are some Do's and Don'ts when compiling a CV:

Do        Always use your portfolio when preparing a CV, both for the purpose of accuracy of information and to select the most relevant material to suit the purpose.

Do        Constantly refer to the job description when preparing the CV, picking out key words that act as clues to identifying the qualities being sought.

Do        Have the CV professionally typed or use a word processor.

Do        Keep the content concise and grammatically correct; have it proof read if possible.

Do        Retain a copy for your own reference and as preparation for any interview that might result.

Don't      Forget to provide your referees with a copy of the CV.

Don't      Prepare your CV in a rush at the last minute. Work on it a few days before the submission date and read it several times. Get a colleague or friend to read it and ask their honest opinion.

*Don't*    Disguise the true facts or tell lies: the outcome could be serious for your personal and professional reputation.

## Diaries, journals and logs

Keeping records by using diaries is probably the most frequent system of recording information and is to many people synonymous with the keeping of a log. Often used on a daily basis, it is a method that requires a certain amount of self-discipline until it becomes a habit or part of one's daily routine. The journal approach is slightly different from that of the diary or log in that it tends to be written less frequently, perhaps weekly, and may take the form of narrative, whereas the log is more a short note or comment. All these systems of record-keeping can be adopted easily without the use of specific documentation or stationery. For the student, a simply daily note of a significant learning event, a valuable experience, a piece of new information or carrying out a new skill might be all that is necessary. The nurse supervisor would likewise record a good learning opportunity provided, the result of a specific patient-centred teaching activity and such things as the student's declared and observed needs and expectations that day. Nurse teachers are not always good at putting into practice what they preach. Having advocated the keeping of a diary or journal to the students and qualified nurses they may then omit to develop the practice themselves, not out of neglect or laziness but because they believe they can readily act upon or recall, when necessary, that which ought to be recorded. The teaching session that was a great success, a student-directed debate that was a total flop and the group discussion that got out of control: each of these situations, should they have happened to a teacher, would probably be remembered at some future date and avoided or modified if necessary. Recording a brief note at the time each happened is perhaps more than just keeping a record — it affords the teacher a second opportunity to reflect about the situation and its circumstances. This is equally applicable for the student and the qualified nurse.

## The nature and purpose of reporting

### Accuracy of reporting

Accurate reporting of factual material and events is not a strong characteristic in most people. When asked to describe in detail the series of events at, say, a motor car accident, research shows that most people will report less than half the facts accurately. At the nurse–patient level can a student transmit accurately that information which is gained by observing a patient's condition or after talking with a patient? A student nurse may report to the ward sister that a particular patient has a chest pain. Apart from the anatomical location this report tells little — there is insufficient information for it to be of any use. More needs to be ascertained of both the frequency or severity of the pain and the quality or subjective description of it by the patient. Very often, the description by a student of something like a pain is distorted by her own perception, experience and threshold of pain. This illustration is given solely to emphasise that reporting must be accurate if it is to be useful. The ward sister who reports to the student's personal tutor that the student is 'always late on duty' when in fact lateness has only occurred three times in the space of a month is perhaps unintentionally presenting an inaccurate account. In some instances this might reflect the subjective feelings of the ward sister towards the student.

## Objectivity and subjectivity of reporting

Reports are usually prepared and delivered for quite specific purposes, such as passing on information, giving advice and making judgements. A report will achieve a higher degree of objectivity if the person compiling it can focus precisely upon the topic of the report and not be side-tracked into other areas. If a nurse supervisor/mentor is to report to the personal tutor or to the student nurse on the progress made in achieving a nursing competency, that, and that only, must be the focus of the report. It is of no consequence that the student is known to prefer another nursing specialism than the one currently being experienced, and any feeling the supervisor may have about the student's political or religious affiliations, for example, must be ignored when presenting an objective analysis of nursing skills acquired by the student.

Dilemmas of this nature are described by Dunn (1984) who feels that report preparation and giving requires very careful planning and thought on the part of the giver, as what the student needs is an educational comment and not a personal view. Almost 20 years ago Long (1976) revealed that while supervisors of students acknowledged that reporting was a vital activity in the overall measurement of progress, they also recognised that their assessment of students was often influenced by factors other than ability alone. Some felt that they were subjectively influenced by particular incidents, others by personality clashes, and a very large number accepted that standards used by supervisors varied immensely. In the same piece of research Long found that half the ward sisters in the survey spent fewer than 10 minutes on the preliminary interview with students. At the end of a student nurse's period of practical experience two-thirds of the ward sisters spent fewer than 30 minutes in preparing the report *and* carrying out the final interview. Subsequent research (Lankshear 1990, Nicklin 1991) reveals that the situation has not improved and, with the introduction of Project 2000, may even have deteriorated. Jowett's (1994) research respondents describe the 'time consuming' burden of student reports as 'time . . . just not there in working hours'.

## Reporting on student nurses

The chapters on principles of assessment and evaluation (5, 6 and 10) deal with the formal aspects of documenting progress and outcomes of student performance, together with the achievements of the course as a whole. What may require a little elaboration is the process of preparing reports and giving those reports to students as part of the curriculum activity. Quite often the student may not acknowledge the report-receiving exercise as part of the educational process: it is sometimes perceived as some form of discipline or counselling activity unrelated to teaching or learning. This misconception may not be all that strange if the reporting session consists of no more than the one-way passage of information or criticism from 'above' to 'below'. For reporting to be an educational activity, it needs to be staged carefully, with both parties being adequately prepared and the 'agenda' of items fully understood by the recipient. To introduce unexpected or unnecessary topics into the reporting session is both unfair and negative in educational terms. Similarly for the student to adopt an uninterested and unresponsive approach as the recipient of a report is not an acceptable response to what should be a rewarding and stimulating interaction for both parties.

Reporting is frequently linked with passing judgements, making comments and levelling criticism. Accepting that these are necessary, the teacher and supervisor might consider also preparing a report when praise and reward is merited: a student may have had a piece of written work published; discharged patients may write to the ward sister praising the care received from a particular student; the ward sister may feel that as a student has contributed significantly to the effective running of the ward or department, she wishes to say thank you and well done! A report that acknowledges and reflects praise is just as much part of the student's training file as a marked examination paper or a study block test score.

Introducing students to the skill of preparing written and oral reports should be done very early in the course — some would say from the first day — particularly if the course employs experiential approaches to teaching and learning. Exposing students to learning situations that require some form of reporting back, whether it is by the individual or as a group, is not difficult to engineer. Reinforcing successful reporting will give the student confidence in the future creation of written reports, each subsequent one becoming more proficient. Through identifying with the need for preparing reports and refining the skill to a high level, the student will have attained a valuable communication tool. Although it can be practical within the assigned work of study periods, its real value will be seen at the practical level, where accurate and objective reporting may influence the type of care the patient receives. The nurse supervisor must ensure that the student practises frequently.

*Receiving reports*

Far from being a passive activity, the receiving of written or verbal reports requires a high level of skill. If a student or any member of the care team has become proficient at preparing and delivering reports, she will quickly become apathetic to the whole process of keeping records and passing on information unless her reports are acted upon in some way. The role of the recipient is to interpret or analyse the report and plan or implement a response, with or without the assistance of the person who compiled the information.

For example, following a meeting of the students' representative committee, its chairman may have prepared a report about the unsatisfactory arrangements for students gaining community experience. How should the course tutor receive such a report, and what may be the appropriate responses? Receipt of the report ought to be acknowledged immediately by the teacher and an indication given of how soon a response to the report can be expected. This procedure should be carried out by the teacher in a calm and professional manner, despite any potential for irritation or annoyance. When a detailed reply to the students' reports has been prepared the teacher may wish to attend the students' representative committee in order to present her reply 'live' and answer any further questions that may arise. Such an approach is both purposeful and professional, showing that students' feelings and opinions are not only respected but also taken seriously.

Where reports are received with bad grace and treated in a contemptuous manner, the result is almost certain to be a total breakdown in effective communication, with the student being the loser, irrespective of who was to blame. Students are frequently asked to report upon the practical experience they have received on a ward or department. If a report is less than complimentary about one of the wards and its staff, how may the ward sister receive such a report? Again the report should be received with good grace and treated seriously. It may be that it is an isolated critical report that is unsupported by other students who have been on the ward. If this is the case, it should be noted and replied to in a courteous and objective way, with copies to the personal tutor and course director. Where subsequent unfavourable reports are received from later student attendances, the ward manager must then begin to carry out in-depth investigations and problem identification.

## Using recording and reporting to produce student profiles

Despite the wide range of measuring devices used to assess the level of attainment of the student and the degree to which competency is being achieved, there is still much about the student that either remains undiscovered or goes unrecorded. In practice when a learning objective has been achieved, it is ticked off a list; the score from a written examination is recorded on the student's file. However little is known about how the student felt when attempting to achieve the objective or what personal motivation led to reaching a high score in an examination. Progress reports completed by the student's supervisor following a period of practical experience tend to focus on what has been achieved or not achieved; very rarely is there any comment on why and how goals were reached. Schools and colleges tend to use measuring devices that are determined by the subjects on the curriculum, argues Law (1984), which unfortunately does not help teachers to know more about their students as individuals. Some of the recording and reporting systems described earlier in this chapter will undoubtedly collect and transmit substantial amounts of information about individual students, but much of the data will be discarded or ignored, mainly because it does not fit neatly into any recordable category in the student's documentation. A wealth of significant material is being lost that could not only help the teacher and practical supervisor to better understand the student but also plays a key role in curriculum development and evaluation. If a student has a particular aptitude for caring for the elderly or handicapped, will this show as a positive feature in the student's records? When planning a particular student's allocation programme to a whole series of clinical experiences, does it matter if this does not take into account the individual's physical characteristics and skills, intellectual ability, social and cultural traits and personal interests? Perhaps a far more meaningful practice programme could be prescribed if some of these aspects of the student's make-up were considered.

Creating profiles for each student need not be a complex matter: basic criteria that can form the main categories for record-keeping need to be agreed. These may include some of the following:

| | |
|---|---|
| — Motivational needs | What works best for the student? |
| — Achievement expectations | Are these realistic? |
| — Hopes and aspirations | Can these be attained? |
| — Assumed skills | Are these confirmed? |
| — Strengths | Can these be maximised? |
| — Weaknesses | Can these be minimised? |
| — Aptitudes | Can these be exploited? |
| — Personality traits | Are these significant? |
| — Physical attributes | Do they have any relevance? |
| — Apprehensions | Real or imagined? |

The above are just a few examples of the types of information that often come to light through the normal process of keeping records. If a base-line profile can be established at the commencement of a course and then be reviewed at appropriate intervals during that course, the resultant changes in the shape of the profile, considered alongside the formal assessment procedures and outcomes, should provide a more comprehensive and accurate account of the student's progress.

## References

Dunn D (1984) Have you done my report please, Sister? *Nursing Times*, **4** (2)

Jowlett S (1994) *Challenges and Change in Nurse Education*. Slough: NFER

Kenworthy N (1993) *Churchill Livingstone, Professional Portfolio*. Edinburgh: Longman

Lankshear A J (1990) *Double Vision*. Unpublished MA thesis, University of York

Law B (1984) *Uses and Abuses of Profiling*. New York: Harper and Row

Long P (1976) *International Journal of Nursing Studies*, **13** (2)

Nicklin P J (1991) *The Quality of Nurse Education*. Unpublished MBA dissertation, University of Leeds

UKCC (1994) *The Future of Professional Practice*. London: UKCC

# 10
# The Nature and Purpose of Evaluation

The ability of any organism to survive and develop is based on, firstly, the extent to which it can learn from past events and, secondly, the extent to which it is able to adapt appropriately as a result. In essence this is the purpose of evaluation in the present context: to learn from past educational events in the life of a student or a course and to adapt them appropriately to reflect future needs.

Reference has been made to the concepts of reflective practice and critical analysis in earlier chapters (3 and 4). In many respects these two concepts are dependent upon the processes of evaluation and review. Evaluation becomes therefore an integral part of the learning process rather than an afterthought or add on. If the principles of reflective practice and critical thinking can be applied to organisations as well as individuals, it can be argued that the organisation becomes a learning organisation, able to learn from the past and adapt to the future. As the only legitimate purpose for a college of health studies to be in existence is to provide educational programmes for practitioners in order to enable them to provide appropriate contemporary health care, the learning organisation can, and must, learn much from its students' comments on the college's activities.

Evaluation is arguably the least understood and most neglected element of curriculum design and development. Teachers often spend many hours carefully considering course aims, objectives, teaching and learning strategies, and at planning team meetings detailed accounts of content matter, methods of presentation and analysis of resources will be examined. Once these very important issues have been resolved, it is then, and only then, that the planning team will address the topic of course evaluation. All too frequently evaluation can be identified as the afterthought attached to the rest of the curriculum strategy — an optional extra. Lawton (1981) suggests that such an attitude is not unreasonable because it is a fact that issues of evaluation present some of the most difficult problems for curriculum planners.

The term 'evalation' is not difficult to define when the prefix 'course' is used. This clearly discriminates it from anything to do with student assessment, which is sometimes, perhaps carelessly, called evaluation. Although terms such as 'the value of' and 'worth while' immediately come to mind, they need qualifying. Together with an indication of the effectiveness of a course, one must consider its justification and consequences. A course may be very effectively conducted in both its content and teaching, but it may no longer meet the needs for which it was designed: those needs may have changed. Courses in the field of elderly care provide examples of this. The course may produce a very competent and efficient nurse able to give care in the institutional setting of a large hospital, so an evaluation of the course would prove it to be totally effective. However the provision of care for older people now has its focus within the community, and the newly-qualified nurse is ill-prepared to function in this changing environment. A new and radically different course is required.

## Classification of evaluation models

The past 25 years have brought major changes in the field of general education, in most cases backed by government money. During periods of financial restraint, concepts of accountability, cost-effectiveness and value for money emerge as key factors in the development of education strategies. As questions relating to student attainment and teacher competency are raised, it becomes increasingly necessary to measure accurately the outcomes of educational processes. Nevertheless there are very real dangers if the sole criteria for evaluation revolve around issues of accountability and cost-effectiveness. It has already been implied that the failure of an educational organisation to respond appropriately to the needs of its customers, be they students, seconding employers or other purchasers, will result in its extinction. We are warned by Hayward (1979) of the need to counterbalance administrative and mechanical structures within human and organic processes.

In nursing education the ENB needs to be satisfied that schemes submitted for approval contain very specific plans for overall course evaluation and the audit of colleges. The 'Guidelines for Educational Audit' (Holroyd and Crow 1993) are referred to in more detail in Chapter 2. For the purposes of this chapter however, this represents an attempt to establish national evaluative criteria, guidelines and models that colleges of health can incorporate into their curriculum design.

The following classification of evaluation models is one described by Lawton (1981) with some additions from other commentators, and an attempt will be made to identify from this classification those models that may appear compatible with the requirements for evaluating nursing courses.

### The classical experimental model

This model relies heavily on quantifiable outcomes. A course employing the model will have very specific behaviour objectives, which can be readily tested, and is likely to be based upon a cognitive taxonomy of educational objectives, e.g. Bloom (1956). Its name derives from the classical experiment whereby a process of pre-testing, teaching programme, post-teaching and control group comparison was employed. Such a model would have a use in courses that are heavily product-orientated and where qualitative values have low importance. A model of this type is feasible in nursing education where the nine competences of Rule 18(1) of the Nurses, Midwives and Health Visitors Rules Approval Order 1983 (DHSS 1983) are precisely broken down into a large number of individual skills. A complex system of cross-referencing could link each of these skills to a particular behavioural objective, which could then be tested. The result would be an accurate analysis of the number of discrete skills acquired, and therefore behavioural objectives achieved, which could then be totalled to determine the degree of competency attainment. This would then have to be validated against a control group of students on a course that did not use this particular approach. It would seem to be a very mechanistic method of evaluation and loses a lot of its immediate appeal when it becomes apparent that little attention is given to the qualitative values of human feelings and attitudes, factors which are important in a course where the target group is human individuals, i.e. patients/clients.

## The illuminative model

An alternative title for this evaluation model is the anthropological model. In direct contrast to the classical model, this provides for a qualitative account of the course. Empirical data are not sought: the main concern is with description and interpretation based upon observation and interview. The advocates of this model would claim that it provides a much wider perspective of the whole course as opposed to just the measurement of behaviour. Furthermore it would appear compatible with the process approach to teaching and learning where experiential methods are employed. Critics of this model would point at its potential for subjectiveness — too much depends upon the interests and values of the observer. This may be a particular problem where the evaluator is also the course manager or tutor, for role conflict is likely to occur. Before this model can become acceptable to those who would prefer more formal methods, its rules of procedure and the skills required to apply it need to be defined more clearly.

## The briefing decision-makers' model

In this model the evaluator is usually an external agent who is 'briefed' to provide information for decision-makers, so this method of evaluation must be concerned with political issues and perspectives. There is no intent to infer that the evaluator simply produces for the decision-makers the answers or evidence that they are seeking; nevertheless there needs to be an awareness of the purpose of evaluation within the context of the relationship between the decision-makers and the course, and the evaluator must carry out his function according to the 'contract' he has undertaken to fulfil. Three types of evaluation are described by MacDonald (1976):

— *Bureaucratic.* The evaluator functions as a consultant working on behalf of a funding organisation, e.g. a government agency. Information elicited from the evaluation report is intended to be used for policy decision-making.
— *Autocratic.* The evaluator functions as an expert adviser. He reports accurately on the educational merits of a course and expects his advice and recommendations to be accepted and implemented.
— *Democratic.* The evaluator functions as an information service. He collects data, interprets them and then presents them to the decision-makers. No recommendations are offered as part of this evaluation.

Despite the differences in approach and emphasis that these three styles offer, their broad aim is to enable the collection of material and data that will assist decision-makers to make better informed choices.

## The teacher as researcher model

Within nurse education it is common practice for the teacher of a course also to carry out the evaluation or part of it. This approach is advocated by Stenhouse (1975) who sees the teacher as both curriculum developer and evaluator. To function effectively in this dual role, the teacher must be research-minded and apply research findings not only to her teaching but also as part of her evaluation techniques. Again the problems of subjectivity and role conflict must be raised when applying this model and it must inevitably be perceived as self-evaluation on the part of the teacher. A technique increasingly used in the self-monitoring model is that of 'triangulation' (Elliott & Adelman 1976). The teacher, student and observer discuss, analyse and compare their observations of the teaching and learning activity, whether it is a single lesson, a course unit or the whole course.

A modified version of triangulation is often used in nursing courses where the clinical supervisor (ward sister), student and personal tutor (observer) evaluate a period of practical experience undertaken by the student nurse.

## The case study model

In this model a wide range of evaluation techniques is used in order to obtain as complete an account as possible of the whole course or course unit. It will therefore employ both quantitative and qualitative methods, which will include measurement, interviews, observations and the use of questionnaires. Because of its very nature it would normally be carried out by an external agency and will therefore have significant cost consequences. An example of case study evaluation is that of employing an independent research body or organisation to evaluate a course or component of a course, which may be appropriate when implementing a new scheme or modifying an existing scheme of training. The difference between this evaluation model and that concerned with briefing decision-makers resides not in its process but in its functional outcome. Although the outcomes are presented to decision-makers, the case study is not necessarily commissioned in order for a decision to be made. It is more likely to be employed to confirm or support a decision that has already been taken and implemented.

### The reflective practice model

The principle of evaluation is central to the dynamic process of reflective learning and critical thinking. Brookfield (1987) points to the close relationship between:

'problem identification, diagnosis, exploration, action and reflection.'

The main difficulty associated here with evaluation is not that it is considered as an afterthought by course planners operating this model, but that of convincing the student that time spent on the activity of evaluation is time well spent.

Establishing evaluation criteria becomes a shared responsibility between the course organiser and the student. Evaluation and review should be a two-way process (Hawkins & Shohet 1989), and an essential part of the evaluation process is to evaluate the evaluation process itself.

### Summary

By examining a number of different evaluation models, it is apparent that an educational course as complex as nursing cannot be effectively evaluated using just one model. As was proposed in Chapter 2 for models of learning, an eclectic approach to evaluation is likely to provide a more complete picture for both student and teacher. Whilst educational factors are of prime concern in any nursing course, the political issues of service provision and staffing establishments cannot be ignored. Performance indicators that reflect both quantitative and qualitative measures in input and output terms are increasingly required by purchasing authorities as part of quality assurance programmes.

Whilst fully supporting the expressed need to obtain value for money and accountability in all aspects of public service, it is essential that general managers should recognise that quality can cost money. A more efficient use of that money is always possible, but there comes a point at which efficiency cannot be increased, and consequently any reduction of resources at that point will result in lowered quality. A summary of evaluation models is shown in Table 10.1.

## The process of evaluation — who evaluates?

All the people involved in a course of education, both at the planning stage and during its implementation, ought to contribute to evaluation. The principal participants in any nursing course are the course teachers, the practical/clinical supervisors or mentors, the students themselves and, most importantly, the patients or clients and their relatives. In addition to these main participants,

Table 10.1  A summary of evaluation models

| Evaluation model | Mode of evaluation | Function of the evaluation | Comments |
|---|---|---|---|
| Classical experimental | Quantitative | Measurement of behaviour using precise behavioural objectives | An eclectic approach — does not consider broader course values |
| Illuminative (anthropological) | Qualitative | Description and interpretation based upon observation and interview | Danger of being subjective — role conflict |
| 1 Briefing decision-makers | Both quantitative and qualitative | Bureaucratic: consultant | May be seen as providing decision-makers with the information they require |
| 2 Briefing decision-makers | Both quantitative and qualitative | Autocratic: expert adviser | It is expected that the evaluation results will be acted upon |
| 3 Briefing decision-makers | Both quantitative and qualitative | Democratic: information service | Provides a detailed report without recommendations |
| Teacher as researcher | Both quantitative and qualitative | Dual role of both curriculum developer and evaluator | Use of triangulation ?Subjectivity ?Role conflict |
| Case study | Both quantitative and qualitative | Factual reporting | Expensive if using an external agency; may be used to confirm beliefs |
| Reflective practice | Qualitative mainly but may include quantitative | Provides the foundation for future learning | Is essential for reflective/critical learning to take place |

there are many secondary or supportive individuals who make an indirect contribution towards evaluation, either by being represented on the curriculum development team or through close working relationships with the key course participants.

The remainder of this chapter will discuss the evaluation roles of the teacher, clinical supervisor, student, patient and curriculum development team.

### Course evaluation and the nurse teacher

The nurse teacher is often involved with the course from its conception to its conclusion. As an active participant at all stages, the teacher may be considered to have a subjective self-interest in its success, but in reality, as Biott (1981) asserts, the teacher should not be denied the opportunity to fulfil the role of 'honest broker' on behalf of the organisation, i.e. the college of health. The nurse teacher, despite this self-interest, has or should have a professional desire to participate objectively in the evaluation of the course. Previous experience will tell the teacher that no course is educationally perfect and that constant modification and revision to structure, content and assessment is essential if a course is to be kept dynamic and responsive to students' needs.

There is far more to the teacher's role in course evaluation than self-evaluation questionnaires, important though these may be. It is valuable for the teacher to keep a weekly log of educational activities as the course progresses. Significant occurrences such as successful learning opportunities and experiences or, conversely, unsuccessful teaching strategies should be noted, together with a comment on future action where necessary. This approach is supported by Rowntree (1981) who advises that a record of this type will assist with a more systematic and objective evaluation of the course or its units.

A number of teachers will usually contribute to a particular course; the teacher referred to as having the evaluation role is the person designated to lead or coordinate the teacher/learning activities for a course unit. As part of the coordination function the unit teacher must arrange for all the other teachers involved to participate in continuing group discussion. If each of these contributing teachers is also keeping a log of significant events, the pooling of information and its analysis will provide important evaluation material. The course or unit teacher must also meet the student group for the specific purpose of discussing feelings and opinions about course effectiveness and the group's perception of progress within the course. Inevitably the students will refer to assessments and their outcomes during a discussion on evaluation, and the teacher will need to have some very clear statements to make about the group work. Analysis of course work, whether it is assessed or not, will form part of the teacher's evaluation report.

It may be helpful to the teacher, and eventually to those involved in the total course evaluation, for an evaluation grid to be completed for each course unit, as shown in Fig. 10.1. The objectives on the horizontal part of the grid are just examples, and other key topics can be substituted.

| Evaluation method | Objectives relating to health concept | Objectives relating to nursing models | Objectives relating to nursing process | Course unit objectives summary |
|---|---|---|---|---|
| Teacher, self-evaluation | | | | |
| Teacher's log | | | | |
| Teacher–peer group discussion | | | | |
| Teacher–student group discussion | | | | |
| Analysis of course work — assessed | | | | |
| Analysis of course work — unassessed | | | | |
| Teacher's subjective evaluation | | | | |
| Overall comments and observations | | | | |
| Evaluation summary | | | | |

Fig. 10.1   Course unit teacher evaluation grid

The teacher on any course is also learning. Critical thinking skills and the principles of reflective practice are as important for the teacher to develop and demonstrate as they are for students. In fact given the characteristics of effective modellers outlined in Chapter 4, it could be argued that the failure of the teacher to exercise overtly the skills of reflective practice and critical thinking could render her a less successful teacher on courses that espouse those values. Increasingly teachers as well as students will need to maintain some form of professional portfolio as a lifelong record of professional achievement. An important element in this is the extent to which the portfolio reveals a developing, adaptable teacher who has learned from evaluating past performance.

### Course evaluation and the practical supervisor

Practical experience directly supervised by qualified nursing staff accounts for over 80% of nursing courses and is correspondingly the most difficult area to evaluate. During the course each student may have as many as 12 or 15 supervisors, each working as a nursing specialist in their particular discipline. Learning objectives for each of the practical experiences will have been declared, and the supervisor's role is to provide opportunities for the student to achieve these objectives. No less significant is the supervisor's responsibility to ensure that the objectives are relevant to the experience being provided and that they are achievable within the time scale available. For specific clinical teaching activities the nurse supervisor can use the same evaluation questionnaire available to the nurse teacher, but this may not be advisable as the 'teaching role' of the clinical nurse is that of facilitator of learning through providing the student with effective experiences. A questionnaire that elicits a qualitative response, whilst having the potential to produce essential information of a type that can be used to keep the learning experiences and objectives dynamic, would seem to be most appropriate.

In the same way that the nurse teacher should demonstrate the critical thinking and reflective practice values of the course, so should the practice supervisor. In fact given the aspiration of most students to be clinical nurses rather than nurse teachers, the practice supervisor is likely to be a more effective model of these skills.

Attention has been drawn previously to the status of the student and the inevitable workload that the student has to shoulder. The skilful ward manager will attempt to safeguard the student's educational interests and indeed utilise, where possible, each component of work as a learning experience.

Where systems of quality assurance are in operation at the clinical/patient level, the supervisor and nurse teacher have a mechanism for identifying the students' workload and the amount of time in learning situations. By using *Criteria for Care* (Ball & Gladstone 1984) in conjunction with workload study, a quantitative measure of student activity can be ascertained. A specimen data sheet showing students' workload and teaching/learning time is shown in Table 10.2, together with an analysis of specific activities.

Table 10.2   Comparison of learner time spent in different activities

| Activity | Hospital 1 | | Hospital 2 | |
| --- | --- | --- | --- | --- |
| | Time spent (min) | % of total | Time spent (min) | % of total |
| Communicating with patients | 5180 | 5.3 | 3690 | 5.9 |
| Patient hygiene | 19210 | 19.8 | 13420 | 21.5 |
| Medication | 5390 | 5.5 | 4060 | 6.5 |
| Charts | 5790 | 6.0 | 4230 | 6.8 |
| Communicating with relatives | 390 | 0.4 | 320 | 0.5 |
| Housekeeping, cleaning | 4030 | 4.1 | 2220 | 3.5 |
| Serving food and drinks, clearing away | 3960 | 4.0 | 3360 | 5.4 |
| Errands | 1070 | 1.1 | 880 | 1.4 |
| Unoccupied | 5460 | 5.6 | 2110 | 3.4 |
| Ward reports | 5440 | 5.5 | 3350 | 5.4 |
| Private study | 950 | 1.0 | 760 | 1.2 |
| Tuition | 1290 | 1.3 | 45 | 0.26 |

Just as the nurse teacher discusses the course progression with students and other teachers, so can the nurse supervisor. At ward team meetings the staff can review student progress, monitor the effectiveness of ward teaching programmes and identify learning problems met by students. At the end of each student's practical ward experience, the supervisor must endeavour to ascertain the student's perception and appraisal of the learning environment that the ward has provided, particularly from a health promotion and nursing skills viewpoint. During the length of a course unit or module, the nurse will have undertaken the supervisory role for a number of students and should therefore be able to reach informed conclusions. It ought to be possible to construct an evaluation grid for each course unit, to be completed by the nurse supervisor for submission to the curriculum evaluation team (Fig. 10.2).

The main purpose of the evaluation grid is to assist the nurse supervisor in determining whether the practical experience is fulfilling the student's needs in addition to the course requirements. Again the topics referred to on the horizontal axis of the grid are the author's preference, and other topics can be introduced.

## Course evaluation and the student

The student nurse is the main subject, centre of focus and sole purpose of nurse training courses. Is sufficient attention paid to her opinions, observations and criticisms of the course in terms of its content, application and assessment practices? Certainly there is an increasing tendency to consult students as part of the process of course evaluation, which may take the form of group discussions, the completion of questionnaires and involvement in curriculum development and review.

It is now common practice for each student group to have a representative and for these representatives to meet at frequent intervals as a students' council or representative committee. One of the committee's main functions should be that of course review and evaluation, but in order to discharge this responsibility adequate advice and guidance are necessary. Without wanting to restrict students to narrow areas of comment, it is necessary to focus attention on relevant issues directly related to the curriculum. Although concerns about residential accommodation, hospital canteens and recreational facilities are important to some students, and need to be debated, these should not impinge upon critical discussions of course progress and satisfaction.

Whilst the student representative committee is a formal body for gathering information relative to course evaluation, Hopson & Scally (1981) point out that informal feedback by way of casual comments from students cannot be ignored. The reported throwaway remark or overhead comment is often significant and a useful adjunct to data that are more formally collected. If students feel that they are a part of the course and its development, sharing in the ownership, they will not only work hard at making it a success but will also seek to criticise its shortcomings whilst also praising its strengths. Students learn better when they feel that they have some control over the learning situation, claim Stanton et al (1980) in their work on courses for the development of social and life skills, an area of study not dissimilar to nursing.

Failure of the college to adequately address real student concerns and anxieties will not only result in a diminishing uptake of places for courses but may also lead to students seeking other, perhaps more destructive (to the college), methods of putting their point across.

Student nurses therefore have not only the right to participate in course evaluation but also a responsibility to do so — a responsibility on behalf of those who follow on subsequent courses. Because students are involved in all aspects of the course, they should contribute to providing information with which to evaluate all components of the course.

Questionnaires are a popular way of eliciting opinion, both objective and subjective, about experiences undertaken in the practice setting and its associated study periods i.e. study block or study days. When questionnaires are to be used, it is necessary to choose an appropriate time and place for their completion, and if questionnaires are to have any merit, they must be addressed in a considered manner by the students, who should be free from constraints of time. It is futile therefore to expect an evaluative questionnaire to have any worth if it is introduced to the students at the end of an allocation with the instruction 'Before you dash off can you fill this in? It will only take two minutes. Thanks.'

In addition to the questionnaire technique, evaluation can consist of one-to-one discussion between the practical mentor and student or in trios with the addition of the nurse teacher. If more than one student is undertaking practical

Key topics for evaluation

| Evaluation method | Health concepts | Nursing theory/models | Nursing process/skills | Other key topics |
|---|---|---|---|---|
| Questionnaire — self-evaluation | | | | |
| Quality assurance analysis — student activity | | | | |
| Peer discussion | | | | |
| Student interviews | | | | |
| Analysis of learning objectives | | | | |
| Analysis of student progress reports | | | | |
| Supervisor's comments, subjective evaluation | | | | |
| Evaluation conclusions and proposed actions | | | | |

Fig. 10.2   Nurse supervisor's unit evaluation grid

experience on the ward or clinical area, it should be possible for students to discuss between themselves the value of the experiences they have received and participated in. Student diaries or journals may be a valuable aid to evaluation, particularly when considering a period of a number of weeks — it is all too easy to base one's judgement on the most recent experiences whilst forgetting what happened in the early weeks of a practical placement.

## Course evaluation and the patient

This aspect of curriculum evaluation is rarely if ever used, and therefore very little information about it is available. Perhaps the problems inherent in conducting such an appraisal are too numerous and complex ever to allow it to become a regular feature of course evaluation. Nevertheless it must be recognised as an ideal to work towards and should be advocated to course teachers and practical supervisors for serious consideration.

Some health authorities are adopting policies designed to offer all patients and clients 'a personal service' in a positive attempt to increase consumer satisfaction. Colleges of health studies working with care providers, where the provision of a personal service is given high priority, must build the concept into all course curricula, and the selective application of appropriate nursing models using the nursing process is an essential component in each curriculum strategy.

The quality of care given to patients can be measured by using such tools as Rush Medicine or its anglicised counterpart, Monitor, together with *Criteria for Care* (Ball & Goldstone 1984). Consumer satisfaction is even more difficult to assess than quality of care; the only guide that most health authorities have is the number of complaints received from patients, ex-patients and relatives in contrast to the number of 'thank you' letters. An attempt to measure patient satisfaction has been conducted by UMIST (1985); however this survey sought to cover all the aspects of a stay in hospital and only a small proportion of the questionnaire related to nurse–patient activity.

Perhaps nurse teachers and practical supervisors could, with the help of patients, design a questionnaire that might be relevant to a student nurse's interaction with and service to her patients. If a survey involving patients is being planned, it should be remembered that the approval of the authority's ethical committee must first be obtained.

More recently the criteria established by the Department of Health in the Patient's Charter, an adjunct to the Citizen's Charter, indicate a continuing move towards a consumer-orientated service. Many purchasing and providing authorities are using these criteria as a basis for their own charter statements, and these criteria are increasingly forming the basis for evaluating educational and training provision — inevitable if policy that determines care provision is linked with education and training strategies.

As patients become increasingly involved in their own care an take and interest in health promotion and maintenance, it is feasible that they could play a more positive role in the student nurse's learning experience. When patients can understand the workings of a model of nursing and the nursing process, they should be able more readily to appreciate the student's educational objectives and assessment requirements.

Regrettably at the moment, only indirect indicators such as quality of care measures and patient satisfaction survey can be used as pointers towards course evaluation.

## Evaluation curriculum development team

Nurse education/training courses are very complex structures. During the period of the course the student may progress through a number of course units, participates in a large range of clinical/practical placements, is supervised by as many qualified nurses, receives teaching inputs from a variety of nurse tutors/clinical teachers and at the same time provides a service for patients and clients. Very few vocational courses can make so many demands upon the student and indeed on those who contribute to the student's learning experiences. If the course is considered to be complex, how much more so is its evaluation? The roles of the teacher, practical supervisor, student, external agency and patient are all considered to contribute to course evaluation, and representatives of these course participants will probably be included in the curriculum development team. In the absence of any formal external evaluating body other than the ENB it would seem appropriate that the team that designed, introduced and developed the course should also process its evaluation. Negative aspects of this arrangement are offered by Heathcote *et al* (1982) who suggest that the evaluator is already committed to the success of the course and that there could well be a tendency towards self-justification. Although they are talking about the single evaluator, the accusation could apply equally to a group. Whilst acknowledging the possibility of self-justification, more attention must be given to the benefits that accrue from the curriculum development team carrying out the evaluation.

Curriculum development and evaluation must not be carried out in isolation or separately from each other — there is a close relationship between the two. This is recognised in a definition of evaluation suggested by Butler & Vaile (1984), which consists of two components: firstly, 'the setting of objectives and standards that act as indicators of how things should be done' and, secondly, 'the appraisal of how things actually are done in the light of set objectives and standards'. The curriculum development team can and should fulfil both roles of development and evaluation. Even more importantly, once an evaluation has been carried out there is the need and will to act upon the evaluation outcomes. This is clearly the function of the curriculum development team and is a responsibility that cannot be devolved to anybody else. This assertion is supported by James (1983) who advocates that those who need to learn from evaluation are those who plan, manage and teach the curriculum.

As curriculum studies become an increasingly significant subject in colleges of health, it is essential that all staff engaged in course delivery develop the skills necessary to contribute to curriculum development: it is a vital developmental requirement in the management of nurse education today. In fulfilling the role of a nurse teacher it is essential that the individual must, in addition to participating as a key member of the development team in relation to curriculum evaluation, be an adviser and resource on all curriculum matters, particularly within the realm of his or her own clinical or subject expertise. In the same way that many clinical skills that were considered to be 'extended role' are now part of the core roles of nurses, the work associated with curriculum development must also be considered as core work for nurse teachers. It is increasingly likely that short 'secondments' to curriculum design projects will form an increasing part of the nurse teachers' work.

The feedback from evaluation forms an important basis for college decision-making. Where a college has a marketing function, it is essential to use evaluation material as positive promotional material, locate courses on a 'product life cycle' and allocate the appropriate resources from the college to particular activities.

Employers and purchasing organisations increasingly have their own approach to evaluation, as separate and distinct from that of the college. Some colleges use a 'first destination employer' evaluation process to capture the views of employers of the college's students, essential information for both student and college.

A number of different models exist for monitoring evaluation material. Increasingly, whilst this material continues to fuel the agenda of course management teams, other bodies within the college also have an interest. These include the senior executive officers of the college, the academic standards monitoring team and the college's academic board. Because the membership of course management teams will reflect those groups involved in different evaluation areas of the course unit, they can not only verify the overall evaluation report but also give their commitment to the actions decided.

An evaluation summary of each course unit may be represented by the grid shown in Fig. 10.3.

Equally as important as receiving evaluation data is the dissemination of proposed actions or curriculum modifications in response to the data. The team must ensure that its decisions on curriculum change are based on wide consultation and are widely publicised to both students and course participants.

## Summary and conclusions

The subjects of assessment and course evaluation are, with very few exceptions, dealt with in educational textbooks as separate items and indeed in separate chapters from the other elements of the curriculum. Although this is understandable for purposes of clarity and discreteness, it does tend to isolate them from what should be a holistic approach to the description of curriculum design and development. Whilst criticising this tendency for authors to compartmentalise the various components of the curriculum, the authors are very conscious of having done this in the structure and presentation of these chapters.

Both assessment of student attainment and course evaluation must be seen as integral features of any course and not mere adjuncts to the content and teaching/learning strategies. At each stage of course design and planning, conscious effort must be given to build in appropriate assessment procedures

| Evaluator | Key curriculum components | | | |
| --- | --- | --- | --- | --- |
| | Health studies | Models of nursing | Nursing process | Others |
| Tutorial staff | | | | |
| Practical supervisors | | | | |
| Student group | | | | |
| External group | | | | |
| ENB Education Officer | | | | |
| Patients/clients | | | | |
| Identified problems/ issues | | | | |
| Proposed solutions/ actions | | | | |

Fig 10.3   Summary of course unit evaluation

and devise mechanisms for evaluating the outcomes in relation to the course unit goals and objectives. Child (1986) goes so far as to suggest that an evaluation strategy ought to be outlined before the course content and its application is formalised. This becomes imperative where assessment and evaluation are more than just a summative appraisal of the student's overall attainment and the terminal conclusion of the course's worth.

It cannot be denied that carefully structured assessment and evaluation strategies are very time consuming for all concerned, from the student to the curriculum development team, but they should be viewed as an economic investment that enables a course to be dynamic and responsive to the needs for change where necessary. What appears to be irrefutable is that courses in the future will find it extremely difficult to survive if they do not have as an integral feature assessment and evaluation strategies that are consistent with the goals and competences that the courses seek to achieve.

The learning organisation needs evaluation material of all kinds if it is going continually to adapt to new circumstances and events and avoid extinction. As constituent parts of the organisation, individual teachers, students and supervisors are also dependent on this information.

## References

Ball J A & Goldstone L A (1984) *Criteria for Care*. Newcastle: Newcastle Polytechnic

Biott C (1981) In Smetherham D (ed) *Practising Evaluation*. Nafferton Books

Bloom B S (1956) *Taxonomy of Education Objectives*. Harlow: Longman

Brookfield S (1987) *Developing Critical Thinkers; Challenging Adults to Explore Alternative Ways of Thinking and Acting*. Milton Keynes: Open University Press

Butler J R & Vaile M S B (1984) *Health and Health Services*. London: Routledge and Kegan Paul

Child D (1986) *Psychology and the Teacher*. London: Cassell

DHSS (1983) *The Nurses, Midwives and Health Visitors Rules Approval Order 1983*. London: DHSS

Elliot J & Adelman C (1976) *Innovation at the Classroom Level*. Milton Keynes: Open University Press

Hawkins P & Shohet R (1989) *Supervision in the Helping Professions*. Milton Keynes: Open University Press

Hayward C (1979) *A Fair Assessment — Issues in Evaluating Coursework*. London: Council for the Education and Training of Social Workers

Heathcote G et al (1982) *Curriculum Styles and Strategies*. London: FEU

Holroyd D and Crow S (1993) *Guidelines for Educational Audit*. London: ENB

Hopson, P & Scally M (1981) *Lifeskills Teaching*. Maidenhead: McGraw-Hill

James M (1983) Course evaluation and curriculum development. *Nursing Times*, **10** (8): 83

Lawton D (1981) In Gordon P (ed) *The Study of the Curriculum*. London: Batsford Academic

MacDonald B (1976) In Tawney D (ed) *Curriculum Evaluation Today*. London: Macmillan

Rowntree D (1981) *Developing Courses for Students*. Maidenhead: McGraw-Hill

Stanton G P et al (1980) *Developing Social and Life Skills*. London: FEU

Stenhouse L (1975) *An Introduction to Curriculum Development*. London: Heinemann

UMIST (1985) *What the Patient Thinks — A Survey of Patients at Three Lincolnshire Hospitals*. Manchester: UMIST

# 11
# Validation

The value of an award or qualification lies in its promise that its possessor has learned to do something that he or she would otherwise be unable to do. The worth of that qualification inevitably lies in the reputation of the awarding body. In order to protect that reputation, an awarding body such as a university must assure itself that any course it is invited to accredit is of sufficient standard to warrant the trust of those who apply to the course and those who subsequently employ its graduates. The Committee of Vice Chancellors and Principals defines validation thus (CVCP 1987):

> Validation is a mechanism for quality assurance; the process whereby a programme of study, its assessment, and the staffing and resources available for the programme are judged to be appropriate to lead to the qualification offered,

and the ENB in its 1993 *Regulations and Guidelines* offers the following definition of validation:

> The process of making judgements about professional, vocational and academic programmes which may lead to a recognised award. This recognition will include meeting criteria reflected in the rules and regulations of the participating bodies.

Before the commencement of a new programme, the decision must be made as to whether the proposals can be delivered in practice in such a way that the students will indeed learn effectively as a result of their exposure to the programme.

In order to practise as a nurse in the UK, aspirants to the profession must satisfy the statutory body, the UKCC, that they can demonstrate the possession of the competences specified in the appropriate act of parliament (DHSS 1983). In their turn institutions offering programmes of nurse education have to be approved by one of the National Boards who seek to assure themselves that the institution is fit to deliver the given programme. This process of *professional* validation has been ongoing since the appellations 'nurse' and 'midwife' were defined in statute.

Whilst courses offered by schools and colleges of nursing have always had *professional* currency, they have traditionally lacked *academic* recognition. In the mid-1980s registered nurses applying to a university to study for a degree were required to undertake the complete programme, no credit being offered in recognition of their RN status. It was then a significant advance when the Council for National Academic Awards (CNAA, now no longer in existence) first agreed that the three-year training equated to the first six months of a degree course and stated its preparedness to grant exemption accordingly. It is furthermore salutary to record that by 1993 the advice offered by the UKCC concerning the recognition of the same course of preparation was that it should be normally worth a full year of a degree (120 Credit Accumulation and Transfer Scheme — CATS — points). This should indicate the complexity of the discussions to be had in the absence of a body of case law and precedent.

One of the key intentions of the reforms inherent in *Project 2000 — A New Preparation for Practice* (UKCC 1986) was that this lack of academic recognition should be addressed. Colleges of nursing and midwifery were to form close relationships with institutions of higher education and the new three-year course pitched at diploma level — defined as two years of a degree course. For the first time teaching and clinical staff concerned with the education of nurses were to offer their courses for academic scrutiny by a university, in addition to having them professionally examined by the ENB, a process termed joint (or conjoint) validation. (The subsequent negotiations were complicated by the fact that many universities had not previously offered an undergraduate diploma qualification.)

The desire for academic recognition was not restricted to pre-registration education. Once alight the blaze spread to all programmes, fuelled by the demands from registered practitioners that their own pre- and post-registration qualifications should receive equivalent attention. Increasingly then, professional programmes of study offered by colleges and faculties of nursing and midwifery are subject to this joint validation process.

The management of a conjoint validation is a complex process, and involvement in it can be confusing in the extreme. A conjoint validating panel can consist of up to 20 members representing the validating university and the educational and service wings of the profession, all of whom come to the exercise with their own special prejudices, interests and values.

### An overview of the validation process

Whatever the unique hallmarks of the institution, the complex process of turning a concept into a successfully validated programme is broadly identifiable from the following description, the steps of which are summarised in Fig. 11.1. Good management of the process calls for application of the principles of project management, and an exploration of the use of project management software such as Microsoft® Project might prove illuminating.

In the first instance a college is required to notify its intention to run the course. This request for 'approval in principle' will require the college to demonstrate the existence of a market demand for the programme and the possession of the resources to mount the course. It will also alert the validating bodies to the need to identify panel members and set a date for the course validation.

Preliminary discussions with
  commissioners of course:
  Identification of training issues
  What will it look like when it's done?
Read appropriate course outlines and
  validating body requirements
Identify programmme development team
  — nominations from senior managers
Arrange meeting of group
Visit other centres offering course
Write outline of course aims
Return to commissioner(s) to check that
  outcomes meet requirements
Discuss with head of department:
  Identify course teacher(s)
  Identify practice placements
Prepare and submit notification to
  proceed to:
  professional validating bodies
  university or other accrediting institute
Identify staff development issues
Arrange any necessary staff development
Identify costs
Commission update of CVs
  produce individual programme project
  plan with target dates and responsibilties
First meeting of group:
  Present rationale for programme
  Present timescale
  Present overall curriculum framework
  Present any pre-existing core material

Commission audits of practice areas
Service reps and course teacher to
  identify outcomes
Begin submission document
Arrange validation and submission dates
Obtain internal validation date
Arrange internal validation event
Disseminate date of event
Amend project plan
Subsequent meetings of group:
  Modify and adopt outcomes
  Decide mode of delivery
  Devise valid and reliable assessment in
    accordance with any available
    guidelines
  Adopt suitable practice placements
Collect placement audits
Identify dates of course
Identify location of course
Ensure and book teaching accommodation
Ensure availability of residential
  accommodation where appropriate
Agree plans for preparation of mentors
Submit booklist to librarians
Prepare final draft submission 1–3 months
  prior to submission date
Arrange/attend internal
  adoption/validation meeting
Make final amendments to document
Arrange copying and binding
Send submission to accrediting bodies

Fig. 11.1   Programme development checklist

The course development team can then proceed to develop the course, working to a deadline date for the submission of a curriculum document, which will describe the course in detail and in a form that, when completed, will be a blueprint comprehensible to those who will put it into practice. The importance of this document becomes apparent to all involved in the validation event as it encapsulates the thoughts, values, aspirations, resources and implementation plans of the organisation. It is sometimes more difficult to remember that the completion of this document is not the end of the process but the beginning.

Before submission of the course documents to the validating bodies, it is usual for them to be considered by the institution's own academic board or a similar internal validating process. At this point any lack of clarity in the proposals can be identified, and those responsible for its delivery have an opportunity to ensure its smooth operation. This internal procedure ensures that the course is owned at the highest level of college management and acts as a quality control mechanism. It also provides a rehearsal for all who will be at the event proper, and its importance should be stressed to those who have not had a previous opportunity to attend a validation at this level. Following internal validation the course is amended as necessary and is subsequently submitted to the external validating bodies. Unfortunately this does not imply that the development team can relax! The work continues with the preparation of all placement supervisors and assessors. Meanwhile teachers will turn outcome statements into teaching plans, deciding precisely how each outcome will be achieved.

Whilst the internal validation event is a rehearsal for the event itself, it should not be the only one planned. During the sometimes lengthy period between the submission of the document and the visit from the validating team, new issues of detailed interpretation, which might challenge the smooth running of the course, will inevitably arise. A final dress rehearsal or practice validation should take place not much more than one week before the event itself and should have a three-line whip. This gives an opportunity for any remaining weaknesses in the document to be identified by the team who have compiled it and responsibility to be allocated for clarifying and correcting that which is unclear. The obvious questions almost bound to be raised (Fig. 11.2) can be allocated to relatively inexperienced members of the team, leaving the experienced die-hards to 'play the googlies'.

---

Can you describe this course to us?

Can you talk us through the diagram on page . . .?

What features mark this course as being at diploma/degree level?

How will communication skills/needs of ethnic minorities/wound care (etc) be taught so that they reflect diploma/degree level study?

Is this post-registration course accessible to second-level nurses?

How do you intend to meet the needs of second-level nurses on this course?

How will the students be supported whilst on placement?

How have placement supervisors been prepared?

50% of this programme is in clinical areas. How can you ensure that this will be at diploma/degree level?

What role will a second-level nurse play in teaching and assessing at diploma level?

Can you assure us of the reliability of your practical assessment strategy?

Are all of the books you believe to be essential reading in the library?

How well does your library service support a student who lives in (name a village in the most remote corner of your area)

---

Fig. 11.2    Questions frequently asked at validation (no money back guarantee can be issued)

## The validation event

Finally there dawns the day of the validation visit. Normally the panel will consist of a course panel of university staff, one or more officers of the ENB and members of the Specialist Registry with particular expertise in the area of study. The panel will seek to be satisfied as to:

— the course proposal;
— the availability and quality of placements;
— access and recruitment;
— the organisation and management of the institution;
— the financial viability of the course;
— the physical resources available for the running of the course;
— the staff;
— the reputation of the institution.

These are considered in detail below.

### *The course proposal*

A curriculum submission is a promissory document. It states an intention to deliver a programme that will enable participants to achieve the desired learning outcomes. However, as elsewhere in life, there may be gaps between promise and action, between intention and execution. Firstly, the panel will have to decide, on the basis of their reading and the questioning of staff, whether the course itself is fit for purpose. If the students on the course achieve the stated learning outcomes, are these of themselves appropriate? The care of a child with diphtheria may be approached with sensitivity and accuracy, and the planning may indicate that students will be effectively taught how to care for such an individual — but is this skill required? Secondly, there needs to be evidence that the panel have taken a long-term view. (It is sobering to remember that a pre-registration course being developed this year will produce its first staff nurses four years hence and, given five years approval, will still be running in nine years' time.) Thirdly, the panel will have considered the academic level of the course. Do the depth and breadth of learning and the intellectual demands on students equate with other courses of that level in the university. This is one of the most complex questions of all. As Wood (1987) points out, how can you demonstrate that a degree in French 'equals' a degree in chemistry? The literature offers little support. In a document designed to help institutions seeking accreditation for nursing courses, the CNAA stated that level 1 was what was taught in the first year of a degree, level 2 equated to what was taught in the second year of a degree and so on. This was generally felt to be about as informative as a dictionary definition of disestablishmentarianism as 'a movement committed to disestablishment'! As a proportion of the first Project 2000 diploma level courses were taken to universities with no tradition of offering nursing courses, the experience of some colleges was that this establishment of academic level was an onerous task. With the formation of reference points and the increasing experience of both validators and validated, the exploration of level should become an increasingly smooth process.

The delivery of professional nursing courses is dependent upon a partnership between education and service. Thus curricular submissions, whilst requiring clear project management, cannot be written by an individual in a back room but must be developed with the full involvement of the teachers and clinical staff who will teach, support and assess the students. Only thus can a course be said to be relevant and its content appropriate to contemporary care delivery. Validators will require evidence that such collaboration has in fact taken place.

Those charged with the assessment of the worth of the course will then seek to satisfy themselves of the degree of dissemination of the information. The delivery of a vocational course is a complex undertaking. There is no point in teachers knowing how the course will be delivered if the manager of an area receiving students has no information as to what they know when they arrive and what they are to learn whilst on the placement. All involved in the course must understand its overall shape and what is required of individual teachers and mentors.

Questions are likely to be asked about the curriculum model. This term is used to describe two different concepts with the result that discussion, even between experienced educationists, can be confusing in the extreme. In its first sense it is used to describe a logical process of course design. After 45 years the model devised by Tyler (1949) continues to pose the pertinent questions:

— What educational purposes should the school seek to attain?
— What educational experiences can be provided that are likely to attain these purposes?
— How can these experiences be effectively organised?
— How can we determine whether these purposes are being attained?

Whilst this model is complete of itself, others have prefaced the process with an explicit requirement to carry out a 'situational analysis' (Nicholls & Nicholls 1978, Skilbeck 1984). At the present time such an analysis of the context of health sector education might highlight the increased scope and volume of day surgery, the reduction in junior hospital doctor hours, the implications of Changing Childbirth and the ramifications of the NHS and Community Care Act. Not only should the present situation be analysed but an attempt should also be made to future-gaze, for the lead time in education, as indicated elsewhere, is lengthy.

The other sense in which the term 'Curriculum Model' is applied relates to the shape of the course itself. Consider for a moment a student commencing a modularised pre-registration training on a course put together totally at random (Fig. 11.3). Such a course is clearly nonsense for the following reasons:

— There is no defined focus, with concurrent modules dealing with different client groups.

— There is no logical progression nor recognition that some things have to be taught before others: for example anatomy and physiology are a prerequisite of pharmacology.
— There is no sense of direction.

The curriculum framework should clearly set out the principles for organisation of material to prevent just such a descent into chaos. The framework should provide shape and logic to the vast amount of learning that should take place during the course. Many curricula in nursing courses use a health–illness continuum as a framework, the focus of subjects initially being the 'normal' individual, while the acutely ill, the critically ill and the chronically ill or disabled provide the focus in subsequent parts of the course. Another approach is to use a developmental model, beginning with childbirth and the care of children and showing progression through the age groups until the spotlight in the later stages of the course falls on the care of older people. Using these client groups as a focus, there are likely to be modules or themes representing the various bodies of knowledge that are brought to bear on the study of nursing: psychology, sociology, ethics, etc.

The level or depth of knowledge or skill required is a further consideration, and here various taxonomies are used as described in Chapters 2 and 3. The experiential taxonomy is one such means of organising course material and ordering teaching methods and assessments according to an explicit belief about how people learn. Whatever the choices made the programme of learning should be presented as a coherent whole and a rationale offered for the sequencing of content and process.

Courses or programmes are increasingly being presented in modular format. Each module is a stand-alone unit of learning with a specified student workload and a clearly defined strategy for assessing whether or not the learning objectives have been achieved. A given number of credit points is awarded on successful completion of each module. The advantage of

The Random Diploma in Nursing Studies — Year 1

| Term 1 | Term 2 | Term 3 |
| --- | --- | --- |
| Clinical pharmacology | Advanced clinical skills: intensive care | Child development |
| Social policy and the elderly | Epidemiology | The concept of health |
| The child with a learning disability | Normal structure and function | The experience of childbirth |
| Supervision and management | Severe mental illness | Nursing theory |

Fig. 11.3   A random approach to planning

modularised courses is that they allow for some degree of latitude, but validators will wish to be reassured that steps have been taken to ensure that courses are coherent and show progression. In other words, that given the freedom to choose modules, there are constraints to prevent students from concocting for themselves an unsatisfactory 'pick and mix experience' such as that illustrated in Fig. 11.3.

Finally the assessment strategy must be examined. It must assess the outcomes that the course seeks to achieve, and its format must be consistent with the course philosophy and the curriculum framework. Most courses utilise a mixed economy of assessment methods in the recognition that, like the students they purport to examine, they all have their strengths and weaknesses. This subject is dealt with at length in Chapters 5 and 6. In addition to the nature of the assessment in use however, their extent is also likely to be a matter for debate. Universities have their own formulae for the calculation of how much pain students should have to endure in order to succeed. A typical exchange rate might be in the order of 3000 words (or a three-hour exam) per 10 credits. This could total as much as 72 000 words for the achievement of a higher education diploma. Jowett *et al* (1994), in their evaluation of the implementation of Project 2000, recommended that consideration be given to:

> 'the course content and structure. There is widespread acknowledgement that it was over-taught and over-assessed.'

The academic worth of the assessment of practice may well be a subject for heated debate in the course of the validation process, as a well-accepted formula for comparing the two suggests that one hour of theoretical time equals to three hours of practical experience. Given that students of nursing have clear outcomes to achieve in the practice setting and that they are assessed by selected practitioners who have been prepared for their role, it can be argued that an hour spent by a student on a day surgery course (for example), acting as a scrub nurse for six procedures, is at least as valuable as the hour spent sleeping through the last lecture on a Friday afternoon.

Throughout, the integrity and coherence of the course proposal will be examined. Claims made within the course philosophy should be identifiable within the learning outcomes and reading lists and examined in the assessment strategy. Although the course philosophy is rightly one of the first things to be written, at the very end of the course design process, a wise team will return to look at it with a critical if not cynical eye in order to ensure that its aspirational statements are substantiated.

### The availability and quality of placements

Depending on the nature of the course and the number and range of placements that it is proposed to use, placement areas may be visited on the day of the validation event or at some point in advance of this date. Much has been said elsewhere in this book about the quality of the learning environment in practice settings, and all of these factors will be assessed during the visits. In the case of a new course, validators will be interested in whether or not students can achieve the relevant learning outcomes in that placement setting. They will observe care being given at the time of the visit and reach conclusions as to its quality. Additionally, of acute interest are the records of care given and the information about the organisation of care yielded by these. Crucially the visitors will assess the attitudes of staff towards, and knowledge of, the proposed course, the arrangements for assigning mentors and the overall staffing configuration of the placement. Students will be asked about their experience of the placement in order to ascertain whether or not sufficient support is available to permit learning to take place. Furthermore validators will require assurance that placement supervisors and assessors have been represented in the course development process and that all participants are fully cognisant of the knowledge, skills and attitudes with which the students will come to any given part of the course, and the learning which should be achieved during that period.

### Access and recruitment

Validators will question course managers about the mechanisms for recruitment to the course and the nature of the entry requirements, if any. A profile of qualifications and experience required for access may be requested. Increasingly the processes for the assessment of prior learning (APL) and the assessment of prior experiential learning (APEL) must be articulated by the institution. The institution will also be called upon to demonstrate how its equal opportunities policy is operationalised and monitored. Selection is the first assessment in the whole programme and, in the view of many, the most crucial, yet it is often paid scant attention within course proposals.

### The organisation and management of the institution

As has already been argued the submission document embodies an intention. In order to put it into practice, the plan must be communicated to the teachers and mentors who will support the students, to service managers who must know when students are expected on placement, to the finance department who will pay and reclaim bursaries and salaries and to the students themselves who must know when, where and how to access the learning opportunities. In order for this to happen the organisation requires sound information and communication networks. Similarly procedures must be in place for the handling of complaints, the management of misconduct and the management of examination marking, moderation and appeals. It is rightly the concern of validators that the organisation is seen to have good management and administrative systems. Where a course is to be delivered by distance learning methods, detailed arrangements for the two-way transmission of materials is required.

The nature of the relationship between the college of nursing and its higher education partner will be carefully considered. Where colleges of nursing are separate from higher education, a memorandum of cooperation detailing the nature and extent of collaboration will be in existence.

## The financial viability of the course

With the publication of *Working for Patients*, the funding of nurse education underwent a fundamental change. The demand for any given course by NHS trusts and directly managed units is assessed at regional level, and a contract between the regional health authority and the colleges within the region is signed. The institution is required to design and deliver the course, recruit to a specified level and comply with a quality specification. In return money is assured from the regional purse to resource the course.

Alternatively a provider organisation can simply purchase training from a college. In this case a representative of these purchasers of education will have to be on hand to record a commitment to funding the course in its entirety.

Funding must cover student salaries (or a commitment to release staff), teacher and support staff salaries, library books and appropriate journals, and a proportion of the costs of overheads (renting, heating, lighting, cleaning and maintaining the building).

Where university validation is being sought, the costs of registration and examination must be identified, as must payment for access to student sports and union facilities.

## The physical resources available for the running of the course

Most learning requires the support of physical resources of some type and the nature of these is dependent on the type of learning undertaken. Distance learning modes require very little in the way of student teaching facilities, for example, but do require substantial investment in the writing, publication and storage of course materials, in the information technology required to track students, and, in its most sophisticated incarnations, in the technologies for radio and television broadcasting.

Where more conventional means of course delivery are adopted, validators will wish to be assured that adequate space is available for both staff and students. While this appears to be an *a priori* statement, recent changes have put considerable pressures on available accommodation. Traditionally, Schools of Nursing welcomed several intakes of students every year. This had the advantage of small class size, permitted optimum use to be made of placements, and ensured a smooth supply of registered nurses for the parent Health Authority. With the advent of Project 2000, more than two intakes of pre-registration students a year were specifically precluded and institutions found themselves preparing to welcome groups of a hundred or more students. Ironically, although the numbers of pre-registration students recruited has fallen by 30% in the three years to date, in many cases intake size has increased as Colleges have sought to rationalise their educational provision and reduce the number of intakes, usually timed to align with the academic year.

Validators are rightly concerned not only with the quantity of accommodation, but also with its quality. As has been noted elsewhere in this book, basic needs must be met before higher order cognitive needs can be addressed. A student who is cold, hungry and uncomfortable will pay scant attention to a lecture on the epidemiology of heart disease. In addition to determining the degree of student comfort afforded by the establishment, there is a need to ensure that classrooms are equipped with all the impedimenta of education — overhead projectors, black or white boards, televisions and video players. As with most other aspects of validation such matters should be addressed routinely as part of the College's own internal quality auditing mechanisms.

The submission document will contain a list of recommended texts. Those charged with the scrutiny of the document are well aware, however, that the compilation of a list demonstrating that teachers are familiar with the most recent texts in a particular subject area is a relatively easy and inexpensive undertaking. More pertinently, they will wish to ensure that these books and journals are actually located within the library or libraries which students will use. For specialist courses, the provision of a postal library service may be required to service the needs of students in placements far removed from the central resource. As technology advances so do expectations. Access to information has been greatly facilitated by the installation over recent years of library management systems and CD-ROMs. These permit students to retrieve lists of published materials by keying in subject areas, author names, title words or key words contained in abstracts. Ultimately as entire texts become available on disk, more and more space in libraries will be devoted to keyboards rather than bookshelves.

Again, as information technology becomes increasingly commonplace in clinical areas, students are required to acquire skills in the use of these systems. This has led to the establishment of a range of computer hardware and software within learning resource centres which constantly has to be updated to keep pace with developments in this fast changing field.

The assessment of learning also has resource implications. With the advent of modularisation and more flexible access through the development of such schemes as the ENB Framework and Higher Award, systems have to be developed to record the progress of students who may accumulate credit points over a number of years. Methods of assessment may also have implications for technical resource availability as these can involve the submission of audio tape or video evidence of, for example, achievement in the area of communication. It is easy to underestimate the resource implications of one hundred anxious students attempting to make one hundred video recordings within a limited timescale, as the author has found to her cost!

The provision and deployment of these technologies breed the need for yet more, for the security of all equipment, bought largely from public monies, is a legitimate concern of those who sanction their use within programmes.

## The staff

It is suggested that the best guarantee of academic standards is the quality of the staff in both the college and placement area who are responsible for the delivery of the course. Staff must have the right qualifications and expertise at the appropriate level to support students. This means that whilst second-level nurses have much to contribute to the teaching of first-level students, they cannot be deemed to be responsible for it. Similarly graduate teachers are required to contribute heavily towards the theoretical preparation of diploma and degree students. Indeed contained within the UKCC's PREP standards, it is confirmed that teaching will become an all-graduate profession, as proposed earlier, and not for the first time, in the Project 2000 proposals (UKCC 1986). Universities place high value on the engagement by staff in scholarly activity, and validators may well be interested in the publications and consultancy record of teaching staff. For some courses it will be deemed necessary to have input from higher education staff — subject specialists in the 'ologies'.

It cannot be sufficiently emphasised that the details of the staff given in the submission document are vital in the assessment of the course quality. As the National Board for Scotland points out in its advisory document (Beattie 1992):

> 'Quite often, CV data has the appearance of having been scratched together begrudgingly, in haste and with no rhyme or reason to the whole exercise. Yet they are vital in the process of validation for a Higher Education course insofar as they give evidence of the likely ability to staff to manage their course at the appropriate level.'

### The reputation of the institution

The ultimate question to be asked in any validation event relates to the trustworthiness of the institution. Does the organisation have a good reputation with its customers? Validators will look to their own experience, to the views of students, to the teachers themselves and to service staff to determine whether all of these groups are satisfied that other programmes offered have lived up to the promises made in advance. Thus assessors being interviewed during the validation of a critical care course may well find that they are being questioned about their experience of the ENB 998 (teaching and assessing). Was it interesting? Useful? Were they well supported? Did they find it easy to access teachers? Were they able to tackle their own individual problems? Was the library appropriately stocked? Such a conversation can to the uninitiated appear to be part of the social warm-up before the commencement of the real business!

### The experience of validation

Validation is a quality assessment that feels like an unseen examination. Observation of any group of experienced educators preparing for such a meeting leaves no room for doubt that it is an occasion for apprehension. Some steps can however be taken to ensure that surprises are minimised. First of all the logistical details should be flawless. A validation checklist (Fig. 11.4) should ensure that everyone who needs to be there has been invited, that the room has been booked and is prepared, and that coffee and food will appear without further organisation on the day itself. Secondly, the curriculum development team should be as well prepared as is possible. Advice on arranging an informal but rigorous dress rehearsal (Frost & Yerrell 1990) has been given above and more follows. Thirdly, it is useful if all members come equipped with the correct document. As there are likely to be two versions of the complete document in existence — the final draft that went for internal validation and the amended version — it is worth clearly distinguishing between the two by the use of coloured paper or dramatically different covers.

---

- receive date of validation, programme of events and names of panel members from validators
- book rooms — including an ante-room which allows participants to gather for the inevitable waits
- write to validators confirming venue and parking arrangements
- list people to be invited to each meeting
- write to individuals inviting them to the appropriate meeting(s) and lunch where appropriate. Include a tear off slip for reply
- provisionally order refreshments/lunch
- confirm numbers and catering arrangements in writing when attendance slips returned
* compile list of expected attendees at meetings
* prepare name cards for panel
* prepare room with adequate seating and tables

Fig. 11.4    Countdown to validation — a guide for education managers

---

The submitting group will normally have some idea from previous discussion with members of the panel where the areas of concern lie, but there are often panel members without previous involvement whose points of view are unknown. Some effort can be made to identify areas of particular interest to panel members by the judicious use of the institution's literature searching facilities. The validation panel (whose membership may for the validation of a lengthy course may be considerable) will typically come together for the first time on the day of the event to compare their views of the submitted documentation. Consensus is not assured, and it is sometimes apparent that having had limited time to plan the visit, there is not always an obvious clearly defined agenda. Managing conflict between validators is part of the art of successfully responding to questions set.

Any group that has put together a complex course has developed its own identity and dynamics. It is highly likely that members have fought, agreed, argued with and supported each other throughout the process. It is therefore inevitably a traumatic experience for the group to find their work interrogated by strangers who may on the face of it appear to be none too keen on the proposals that the group has worked so hard to compile. The nature of the adversarial process is such that it is easy for the institution being validated to be fearful and correspondingly defensive. At such times it is difficult to remember that the process is one of genuine enquiry in the interests of protecting students, prospective employers and ultimately patients and clients (Beattie 1992):

'Charges levied against validation events include the claims that the process is prescriptive or confrontational or unduly conservative or rests on unspoken assumptions on the part of panel members as to what constitutes a good course. The debate conducted is therefore one of closure rather than of opening.'

Even if this is felt to be applicable in any particular case, strenuous efforts must be made to resist knee jerk defensiveness, which all too often feels to the validators like aggressive obduracy. Challenges may arise as a result of too little information being in the document. It is impossible to represent all the discussion that has taken place during the period of course development. The team must be aware however that what is not clear to the panel will not be clear to those who deliver the course, and therefore all concerns are valid. Sometimes the group will be able to reassure panel members that the information they require is to be found elsewhere amongst the documentation or that the decision that is being questioned is based on sound and rational judgements. Sometimes the group will acknowledge that a point has not been sufficiently carefully thought through and offer to clarify the position before the start of the course. There is a fine balance to be achieved between convincing the panel that the team has carefully considered all the eventualities that might arise as the programme is translated into practice and recognising valid criticism and good suggestions that should be acknowledged with thanks.

Evidence of collaboration with service staff during the planning process is sought by their playing an equal part in the validation event, but experience shows that this participation is difficult to achieve. Groups of highly articulate and passionate clinical staff who have engaged in a heated defence of curricular decisions during the internal validation process have all too often been stunned into silence at the event itself. Sadly but frequently, discussions at validation events rely heavily on the use of technical educational terminology and as such are difficult to access for those who have no views on the relative merits of the proposed taxonomy. A good panel of validators will however make it their aim to elicit information from representatives of all those who will be involved in the course delivery. Compared to the limited information to which the panel has access, every member of the group is an expert in their contribution to the proposed course and should take every opportunity to explain this to the members. As has been pointed out, there are expected questions for which responsibility can be allocated in advance (Fig. 11.2 above).

### The outcome of validation

The result of the enquiry is normally available on the day of validation. The period during which the panel is deliberating is set aside for the curriculum development team to bite their fingernails and think of all the things they should have said when they had the opportunity.

Courses can either be approved, approved subject to conditions and/or recommendations or can fail to meet the requirements. Conditions *must* be met, usually before the course commences. In the case of recommendations the institution is called upon to give serious consideration to the view of the panel but has discretion in relation to the response. It is useful to have in the room a secretary with good shorthand skills to take notes so that the curriculum group can commence work on meeting any conditions set within the timescale indicated.

Whether a celebration or a wake is called for, an opportunity to debrief is advised. In the author's experience this is, wherever possible, best carried out in the local pub.

## References

Beattie A (1992) *Ensuring Quality and Standards in the 1992 Programme.* Edinburgh: National Board for Scotland

Committee of Vice Chancellors and Principals (1987) *University Validation of Courses in the Polytechnics and Colleges Sector.* London: CVCP

Department of Health and Social Security (1983) *Nurses, Midwives and Health Visitors Rules Approval Order*, Cmnd 873. London: HMSO

Department of Health (1989) *Nurses, Midwives and Health Visitors Act Rules Amendment Approval Order*, SI 1436. London: HMSO

Department of Health (1989) *Working for Patients.* London: HMSO

ENB (1993) *Regulations and Guidelines for the Approval of Institutions and Courses.* London: ENB

Frost S & Yerrell P (1990) *Developing Education for the Future Managing the Validation Process.* Sheffield: ENB

Glen S & Jamieson I (1993) The validation event: a critical appraisal? *Nurse Education Today,* **13**: 161–166

Jowett S *et al* (1994) *Challenges and Change in Nurse Education — A Study of the Implementation of Project 2000.* London: NFER

Nicholls A & Nicholls N (1978) *Developing a Curriculum: A Practical Guide.* London: Allen and Unwin

Skilbeck M (1984) *School Based Curriculum Development.* London: Harper and Row

Tyler R W (1949) *Basic Principles of Curriculum and Instruction.* Chicago: University of Chicago Press

UKCC (1986) *Project 2000 — A New Preparation for Practice.* London: UKCC

UKCC (1994) *The Future of Professional Practice — The Council's Standards for Education and Practice following Registration.* London: UKCC

Wood R (1987) *Measurement and Assessment in Education and Psychology.* London: The Falmer Press

# 12
# Developments in Nurse Education

'Change is not what it used to be, and the only safe prediction is that there are no safe predictions . . .' was the starting point of this edition of *Teaching and Assessing in Nursing Practice.* Nothing has changed that proposition in the preceding pages. A chapter on developments in nurse education is therefore descriptive rather than predictive and seeks to describe the terrain rather than prescribe a route in a rapidly changing environment.

For many nurses, doctors, academics and others, the application of market principles to health and education is not only alien but also anathema. Of the increasing number of the population who are dependent on their services, many find the notion of a market in health and education contradictory to their expectations of a welfare state (or welfare society). But what is marketing? Marketing can be defined as:

'the means by which an organisation (such as the NHS) matches its resources (human, financial and physical) with the needs of its customers (the population) in order to meet its objectives.'

This somewhat benign statement only becomes contentious when resources cannot keep pace with demand or expectations. A short chapter on developments in nurse education cannot possibly aspire to analyse or explain how economic, technological, political, demographic and other forces have conspired so sternly to challenge the vast majority of those employed in the business of health and education. For many, Handy's (1994) observation that 'we are not where we hoped to be' rings true. But where will nurse education be at the end of this decade and at the beginning of the 21st century? As 'there are no safe predictions' the author will confine his ambition to merely describing some possible scenarios.

## Marketing health sector education

The definition of marketing used above embraces a range of dynamically related activities or issues known as the *marketing mix*, which provides a useful framework for discussing developments in nurse education. The marketing mix consists of:

— products (and services);
— price;
— place;
— personnel;
— promotion.

### Products and services

Nurse education supplies and provides a range of products and services to a variety of customers and consumers. Distinctions between products and services, and customers and consumers, is not straightforward but is briefly mentioned here because of the significance such definitions have on the business of health sector education. Shostack (1982) argues there are very few 'pure' products or services. Services are typically intangible insofar as they are consumed but not owned. In this respect students could be considered to receive an educational *service* whereas employers are recipients of skilled labour — a *product*. In Chapter 2 a distinction was made between customers and consumers — 'the convention to describe the user of public sector services as consumers . . . the term customer implying direct payment for a commodity or service'. Using this convention students could be regarded as *consumers* and education contractors as *customers*.

Here reside some of the major challenges and tensions for health sector education. A market exists to provide a satisfying exchange relationships — but who shall be satisfied? The needs and expectations of employers, validators, students, statutory authorities, the public and patients are not necessarily the same. Nor is it as simple as 'he (or she) who pays the piper'; the cost of education is increasingly being met by students directly — the consumer is becoming a customer. Also so-called market forces are dynamic and notoriously unpredictable. During the late 1980s concerns about the 'demographic time bomb' spawned slogans such as 'wrap jobs around people — not people around jobs' and resulted in almost heroic efforts to recruit and retain student nurses. The entry gate was widened (but not lowered), courses became more flexible to meet the needs of students with dependent relatives, the long-standing obstacles to enrolled nurse conversion were removed and Project 2000, which would enable nursing to compete for the declining number of young people entering the labour market, was approved. In the mid 1990s we are not where we thought we would be, and many of the policies and practices of the preceding decade show a poor fit to current market conditions, as well may current policy, practice and values during the next decade, the beginning of the 21st century.

One maxim of the market is 'many a company producing high quality goods has gone to the wall because there is no demand for their product'. The issue here is about 'fitness for purpose'. One potentially disabling legacy of nursing and education is the notion of 'highest possible quality'. A more enabling and affordable concept is 'good quality does not necessarily mean high quality, it means a predictable degree of uniformity and dependability at low cost with a quality suited to the market' (Deming 1986).

. . . **Suited to the market**    What can be safely predicted is that the demands of the market in the year 2001 will be significantly different from those in 1991. Possible scenarios described by the Department of Health (1994) include:

— a shift from institution-based care to community care;
— continued expansion of minimally invasive surgery and 'day surgery';
— a reduction in the length of hospital stay and a reduction in the number of acute hospital beds;
— a substantial increase in a range of services and treatments offered by general practice;
— a 'mixed economy' of care providers — public, private and voluntary.

These changes in practice have fundamental implications for education, some of which are already apparent:

— The number of entries into pre-registration education will continue to decline before stabilising. During 1992/93 fewer than 16 000 students entered pre-registration programmes, 45% fewer than commenced 10 years previously. Conversely there will be a continued expansion in the volume and range of post-registration programmes, accurately reflecting the need of providers to skill and re-skill their staff to meet the demands of changing patterns of care.
— Colleges will need to be increasingly responsive and flexible in their provision of programmes. Employers will demand prompt training solutions to their immediate problems. There will be increasing pressure to reduce the length of time required to design, develop, validate and implement programmes.
— the boundaries between professions will become increasingly permeable. Some time ago Peach (1987) observed that 'one of the passages in the original Project 2000 discussion papers excited little debate but has interested me. This was the suggestion that the Common Foundation Programme might form the basis for a common foundation for shared learning with other workers . . . were we to pursue the idea of shared training further there could be pay-off in terms of greater productivity as well as undoubted benefits of greater shared understanding of the common task'. This is an idea whose time has come. The role of the professional statutory body is after all to protect the public, not to preserve redundant professional boundaries.

— There will emerge a 'mixed economy' of educational providers. Consortia of NHS Trusts will increase their capacity to provide vocationally accredited programmes. Independent training agencies and consultancies will increasingly compete with colleges for short course and in-service provision.

## Price

The price that customers pay is an expression of the value that they place on a service or product and reflects their purchasing power or ability to pay. In general terms there are numerous variables that influence price and price variation. In the open market the availability or desirability of a product is more likely to determine price than is the cost of manufacture or provision. The difference between *price* and *cost* contributes significantly to *profit* (or loss). Health sector education is of course 'not for profit'. Consequently, theoretically at least, cost = price.

The challenge for nurse education, as elsewhere in the public sector, is to demonstrate cost improvement, i.e. increased productivity without increasing costs or maintaining productivity at a reduced cost. This fairly simple notion is complicated by the fact that many institutions do not as yet have a sufficiently comprehensive understanding of their real costs or control over their levels of activity. As colleges of nursing have combined with each other or integrated with higher education, costing differentials have become apparent. Clearly if an equitably managed market is to emerge, costs have to be known and understood, the 'nightmare scenario' being that a college will undercut the costs of its competitors to win contracts and then not be able to afford to deliver them. In the meantime its competitors, who realistically costed their services, are out of business — the classic lose–lose scenario.

Cost however is more than price. Cost is also about 'benefits' and 'value added'. These concepts are illustrated by the following examples:

— In comparing the cost (or price) of a programme at a particular institution, issues of reputation and quality emerge. Is for example the course and award of 'Camford University' comparable with that of the equally fictitious 'University of Plumstead'?

— Some colleges, by virtue of geographical location and historical reputation, have first choice of candidates. But what of the inner-city college, which might be less attractive to candidates? A college that has second choice of candidates but returns comparable results at a similar cost could be regarded as giving 'value added', in other words more than was expected, and giving better value than its more prestigious competitors.

— the cost–benefit equation includes consideration of the local infrastructure and economy. A college may have an excellent academic reputation but high residential accommodation costs or may be located in an area that experiences above average crime against property and the person.

During the next few years nurse education will ascend a steep learning curve on issues relating to cost and prices. Furthermore, the source or burden of funding is likely to be reviewed and revised. Earlier it was indicated that funding for post-registration education is shifting from the employer to the employee; it is anticipated that this shift from public to personal funding will also extend to pre-registration nurse education. As nurse education assumes the values of higher education, it might be assumed that it will adopt its funding regime. This option is not unattractive to the exchequer; a shift from NHS bursaries to means-tested grants and student loans could yield savings in excess of £200 million per year (1993/94) — presumably the price that nursing, or more specifically students (and their parents), will pay to become an 'all graduate' profession.

## Place

Place is a key concept in the marketing mix and is concerned with the efficient and effective distribution of services and products to customers. When applied to nurse education the notion of place inevitably leads to a consideration of classrooms, laboratories and clinical facilities, which represents a useful starting point for this discussion. However 'place' is a much broader concept than buildings, as will be reflected as this debate progresses.

Much nurse education estate is located in converted hospital buildings and, according to the Committee of Vice Chancellors and Principals (1994), is 'poorly maintained'. Whilst the author is unaware of a national audit of school of nursing estate, impression and anecdote suggest that health sector education facilities, in the main, compare unfavourably with those in higher education. This is not so much an issue of historical neglect but an accurate reflection of former planning and priorities. When colleges of nursing were managed by district health authorities, they had to compete directly with clinical services for capital developments. It is hardly surprising that a community unit for the elderly or a neonatal intensive care unit might receive funding preference over a library or media resource suite. Colleges are now quasi-independent, managed at 'arm's length' by health authorities and moving towards integration with the higher education sector. This means they have increased control over their planning and priorities. If the money were available (and it's not), should health sector education make a substantial investment in its estate? — probably not. Capital investment, capital charges, leases, loans and maintenance add to costs (price). An alternative scenario is fewer buildings of higher quality that are used more extensively, combined with a more rigorous application of existing and potential technologies and a revision of traditional working practices. But what does this mean? It could mean:

— substantially increasing classroom occupancy levels by extending the 'operational' (not individual) week to include evenings and weekends;
— the further expansion of distance learning methods;
— audio and video conferencing, which reduces the requirement to travel from 'remote' sites and reduces the demand for large and costly 'central' facilities;

— a substantial expansion in home working, employees being linked by electronic mailing facilities;

— more extensive use of the customer's workplace as the venue for training.

None of this is particularly visionary, and some of it is contentious. What is being argued for is fewer and better facilities that are more effectively managed. The costs of nurse education are transparent to its customers·who are unwilling to subsidise wasteful practices that contribute to their own costs.

Place is about customers accessing services and products. Beyond buildings this discussion has so far briefly alluded to workplace-based learning, distance learning and video conferencing, initiatives that take the service to the customers and are constructed for their convenience rather than that of the provider. Other initiatives might include postal or mobile libraries that give students access to not only books and journals but also literature searches, CD-ROM and video material. As organisations become IT integrated, electronic networks will enable computer-based interactive seminars to be used more extensively in the workplace or at home. Some colleges have introduced telephone 'helplines' so that students needing guidance on study, research, assignments or projects can contact a teacher at any time of the day (or night). Clearly there is much more that colleges can do to get their services to their customers — and those who do will survive.

Any discussion on place would be incomplete without a consideration of the European dimension. During the preparation of this book mainland Britain was linked to the continent of Europe by a tunnel, the first physical link since the last Ice Age. But why is everyone so concerned about 'going into Europe'. 'Why', retorts Paul Merton (author and comedian), '— can't we go into Brazil where the weather is better?' The following comments will not address the questions of the Euro-sceptic or the Euro-illiterate; their purpose is merely to assert that Europe presents opportunities and challenges for nurse education. General nurse (adult branch) training has of course been subject to a European Directive since 1979 (77/452/EEC), as has midwifery since 1983 (80/154/EEC). The objective of these and other Directives is of course to improve the provision of health care to the people of Europe. In recent years colleges of nursing, through their higher education links, have started to participate in European Community programmes such as LINGUA (Programme for the Promotion of Foreign Languages Knowledge in the EC), ERASMUS (European Action Scheme for the Mobility of University Students) and COMETT (Community Programme for Education and Training for Technology). Colleges are increasingly participating in educational and clinical exchanges, which is in accord with the aims of the European Union (Article 126), which includes:

— developing the European dimension in education, particularly through the teaching and dissemination of languages;

— encouraging the mobility of students and teachers, by encouraging academic recognition of diplomas and periods of study;

— promoting cooperation between educational establishments.

Getting Europe onto the agenda and into the curriculum is not merely about conforming to Directives but also about making the nursing contribution to a more prosperous, healthier and harmonious Europe (on the latter point the author also notes that this edition was being prepared on the 50th Anniversary of D-Day). But what of the other Europe, the Europe beyond the Union, mainly but not entirely the countries of the former Soviet bloc. Possibly the greater challenge to health sector education is to enable and assist these countries to establish and develop their nursing and nurse education services.

### Personnel

People are simultaneously health sector education's major asset and its most costly expenditure item; consequently they are at the heart of the marketing mix. In short this section will concern itself with *doing things right* — having the right people, in the right job at the right price.

Readers will be familiar with the cliché 'those who can, do — and those who can't, teach'. Whilst there have always been healthy tensions between theory and practice and allegations that teachers were 'out of touch', the credibility of nurse teaching has never before been so seriously questioned. What is different on this occasion is that it is a two-pronged assault from clinicians and academics and that, in part at least, their criticism is contradictory. The concern of clinicians and their managers is that teachers have insufficient clinical expertise and that they are poorly equipped to deal with vocational (NVQ) training. The ENB's (1993) solution is that teachers should be employed in clinical practice for the equivalent one day each week. On the other hand university staff, according to *The Times Higher Education Supplement* (6 May 1994), are more concerned about academic content, assert that nurse teachers are 'trying to run before they can walk' and by implication doubt their ability 'to improve academic standards in [nurse] training'. The RCN (1993) provides a thoughtful and thought-provoking analysis of the conundrum, and concludes that:

— the current system of *task-centred teaching*, characterised by increasingly different roles and simply adding more tasks to existing workloads, is destined to fail;
— a more obvious alternative is *discipline-led teaching*, with teachers specialising in the academic disciplines that contribute to nursing. Whilst this approach firmly links nurse teaching with the wider academic world, it simultaneously dislocates nurse teaching from nursing. In the words of the RCN discussion document, 'by definition "ologists" will gain ascedancy, like cuckoos in other birds' nests'. Consequently this is also rejected as a viable strategy;
— the way forward is through *practice-based teaching*, where teachers are actively based in clinical nursing, nursing research or the management of nursing services, the RCN suggests that it 'might be characterised by a long term employment contract linked with a series of highly flexible,

short term "role/function contracts".' Additionally it believes it imperative that nurse teachers of the future should be graduates in nursing and nursing-related subjects.

Certainly it is crucial that nurse education develops skills required and respected by the market, but just as important is the flexible deployment of those skills. As with other services nurse education has to balance supply and demand. Although the demand for pre-registration programmes may be reasonably predictable, the demand for short courses, in-service programmes and research may fluctuate dramatically and it is this latter group that is becoming an increasingly important market segment for nurse education. Cost-conscious competitive organisations cannot afford to fund 'down-time', those periods when their ability to supply exceeds the demands of the market. One solution is to reduce staffing to a 'core' that meets the predicted needs of the market and to employ contractors or consultants for fixed terms to manage periods of increased or unusual demand, as illustrated in Fig. 12.1.

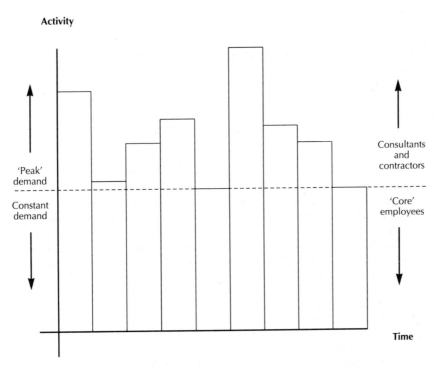

Fig. 12.1    Balancing supply and demand

Organisations that have a relatively small core of full-time workers surrounded by a flexible periphery of contractors and consultants are, according to Handy (1994), employing the 'doughnut' principle, precisely the principle employed by many university research departments, the Open University and the Nursing Times Open Learning Programme. The 'doughnut' principle poses simultaneously a threat and an opportunity for many engaged in nurse education. Certainly it does not mean a job for life, as it is (or was) commonly understood. What it could mean, for those whom the RCN (1993) describe as 'wholesome entrepreneurs', is a flexi-career constructed around a portfolio of activities, which might include part-time packages of clinical nursing, specialist teaching, consultancies, research and publishing. As colleges increasingly attempt to manage fluctuation in workload and respond to market opportunities, demand for 'portfolio workers' will intensify. Portfolio working is also a creative and effective method of managing personal or career transitions. A portfolio may contain 'space' to care for a dependent relative or facilitate the transition from full-time employment to eventual retirement.

### Promotion

Promotion is possibly that element of the marketing mix that the reader could most easily identify with. In discussion the words 'marketing', 'promotion' and 'advertising' are frequently interchanged as though synonymous. In this chapter the author has already suggested that marketing is a comprehensive construct, and similarly it is argued that promotion is not exclusively advertising. The role of promotion to nurse education is:

'to communicate the benefits of the products (and services) and the merits of the institution to existing customers, potential customers and to stakeholders'

and consists of two distinct but complementary activities: advertising and publicity.

**Advertising**    This is the area in which the organisation pays to construct and communicate its message. Advertising is used to promote the organisation's objectives through the mass media, for example by advertising a course, conference or job vacancy in a professional journal or local newspaper.

**Publicity**    Publicity is typically in the form of a news story about the organisation, its activities or its personnel. Publicity is distinct from advertising in that it is not paid for, although there are costs associated with preparing press releases and encouraging the media to use them. Whilst advertising is controlled by the organisation, publicity is managed by the media. For example a college's celebratory message of '100% pass nursing examinations' might become, after further investigation by the media 'poor job prospects for newly qualified nurses'.

When (if ever) nurse education was unquestionably regarded as a 'good thing' and its abilities and performance were undoubted, the need for promotional activities was probably marginal. With the emergence of a managed market, it is evident that nurse education and educational institutions must have a coherent promotional strategy. But a note of caution. The glossy prospectus, promotional pen, clever logo and alliterative corporate slogan do not constitute a promotional strategy and may alienate customers if perceived merely as 'glitz' and rhetoric. If the promotion of the college does not square with the staff or student experience, or is considered to be extravagant or wasteful, healthy scepticism can be converted to a debilitating cynicism. Indeed the most effective sales force are a thousand or more satisfied staff and students who, quite unsolicited, describe the benefits of the institution and its course to their friends. Reputation has a lot going for it. Nicklin's (1991) research on the quality of nurse education revealed that 'reputation was a composite and consequence of all other "quality" factors' and 'the most powerful sentiment expressed, . . . respondents spoke with pride and affection about schools and colleges'.

## There are no safe predictions

In concluding this chapter and this edition of *Teaching and Assessing in Nursing Practice*, it is worth summarising the broad characteristics of nurse education in the future. Whilst 'there are no safe predictions', there are fundamental principles that will shape the education service of the future. The DoH (1994) summarises these; the education service must be:

—  *patient-focused*: developing practitioners who constantly strive to improve the care of patients and clients, their families and the wider community;
—  *practice-led*: rooted in the art and science of nursing, midwifery and health visiting as practical activities;
—  *student-centred*: recognising the individuality of students and harnessing the wealth of experience that they bring to the learning situation, and making programmes accessible, attractive and challenging in terms of both personal and professional development;
—  *equitable*: providing equality of opportunity;
—  *appropriate*: preparing practitioners who are 'fit for purpose', with the knowledge, skills, attitudes and commitment to personal professional development necessary to function confidently, competently and with sensitivity;
—  *effective*: achieving the highest standards whilst making the most efficient use of resources;
—  *responsive*: employment-focused and capable of adapting to changing health needs with minimum disruption and maximum speed, making full use of research findings to inform curriculum design, delivery and evaluation;
—  *collaborative*: securing the cooperation of the major stakeholders to work in partnership, to recognise and to achieve a common purpose and to create opportunities for shared learning with other professions;
—  *accountable*: open to scrutiny, explicable and defensible.

Achieving all of this in a constantly changing and at times contradictory environment poses new challenges and requires new ways of thinking and new ways of working. Kanter (1989) likens this environment to the croquet game in *Alice in Wonderland*. The mallet is a flamingo which frequently lifts its head and faces in another direction just as Alice is about to strike the ball. The ball is a hedgehog, which just at the moment of impact unrolls, gets up and moves to another part of the court, and the hoops are playing card soldiers who, at the whim of the Queen of Hearts, reposition themselves around the playing area. Kanter suggests, 'substitute technology for the flamingo, employees or customers for the hedgehog and everyone from government regulators to corporate raiders for the Queen of Hearts, and the analogy fits the experience of a growing number of companies'. Kanter identifies five characteristics of successful companies (the five Fs); they must be:

— *fast*: have good external antennae, hear what their customers have to say and respond quickly;
— *focused*: know what they do well and are passionate about. They do not try to do everything, or paddle about in someone else's business;
— *friendly*: both to internal and external customers. They don't get caught up in debilitating power struggles;
— *flexible*: and adaptable and find new solutions to respond to new circumstances;
— *fun*: give their workers a 'buzz'; their people look forward to coming to work. Successful organisations take fun seriously.

If nurse education is to achieve its strategic objectives, it will require liberal use of the 'F' words.

## References

Committee of Vice Chancellors and Principals (1994) *Nursing and Professions Allied to Medicine*. Report of a CVCP group. London: CVCP

Deming W E (1986) *Out of Crisis*. Cambridge: Cambridge University Press

DoH (1994) *Nursing, Midwifery and Health Visiting Education — A Statement of Strategic Intent*. London: DoH

DoH (1994) *The Challenges for Nursing and Midwifery in the 21st Century*. London: DoH

ENB (1993) *Regulations and Guidelines for the Approval of Institutions and Courses*. London: ENB

Handy C (1994) *The Empty Raincoat*. London: Hutchinson

Kanter R S (1989) *When Giants Learn to Dance*. London: Unwin

Nicklin P J (1991) *The Quality of Nurse Education*. Unpublished MBA dissertation, University of Leeds

Peach L (1987) *Address to RCN Manpower Conference*, May 1987.

RCN (1993) *Teaching in a Different World*. London: RCN

Shostack G L (1988) How to design a service. *European Journal of Marketing*, **16** (1): 49–63

# Appendix 1
# Glossary of Terms

**Accreditation of Prior Experiential Learning (APEL)**  Non-formal forms of learning acquired, often unintentionally, through life experiences generally, paid and unpaid work and study that may or may not be formally certified.

**Accreditation of Prior Learning (APL)**  A process by which individuals can claim and gain credit towards qualification based on evidence from their past achievements, i.e. formal 'certified' courses.

**Approval**  The outcome of validation, which includes formal confirmation that the institution and the course or programme have been judged to meet requirements.

**Approved institution**  An educational institution that is approved as having met the ENB's requirements for the conduct of courses for nurses, midwives and/or health visitors.

**Assessment — formative**  Continuing and systematic appraisal of a student to determine the degree of mastery of a given learning task and to help the student and teacher to focus on the particular learning necessary to achieve that mastery.

**Assessment — summative**  An assessment of the extent to which a student has achieved outcomes/objectives for the course as a whole, or a substantial part of it, contributing to the grading of a student for qualification for an award.

**Assessor**  An appropriately qualified and experienced first-level nurse/midwife/health visitor who has undertaken a course to develop his/her skills in assessing or judging the students' level of attainment relating to the stated learning outcomes.

**Audit**  Part of the cycle of quality assurance. It incorporates the systematic and critical analysis by course management tutors of clinical placements, in terms of outcomes for students and introduces appropriate changes to that analysis.

**Competenc(i)es**  The ability to perform particular activities to prescribed standards.

**Conjoint validation**    Validation undertaken simultaneously by the ENB and an awarding body in equal partnership.

**Continuing professional development/education**    Those teaching and learning activities, including open and experiential learning, that follow initial education and training and are directed at maintaining and improving the quality of service/care provided. It contributes to the habit of learning, which enables the individual practitioner, the profession and the service to evaluate the quality of service/care and improve it through practice, education, management and research.

**Course/programme**    A number of units of study, the successful completion of which leads to an award.

### Credit Accumulation and Transfer Scheme (CATS)
— *Credit accumulation*: a system whereby individuals can acquire credit that may count towards a professional or academic award.
— *Credit transfer*: a system whereby individuals may transfer the credit they have acquired to another programme or institution.
— *General credit*: a numerical value representing the credit points attached to quantifiable prior learning of an intending student without this being considered in relation to a particular programme of study:
— *Specific credit*: the credit that is directly relevant to an individual student's particular programme of study.
— *Level*: the level of a unit or course as an academic measure of how far that unit or course corresponds to the academic standards required in one of the years of a first or higher degree.

**Curriculum**    An attempt to communicate the essential features of an educational proposal in a form that is open to critical scrutiny and capable of effective translation into practice.

**Indexing**    A formal administrative procedure that records that a student is eligible for and has entered upon a course of study that may lead to registerable or recordable qualification or the Higher Award.

**Mentor**    An appropriately qualified and experienced first-level nurse/midwife/health visitor who, by example and facilitation, guides, assists and supports the student in learning new skills, adopting new behaviour and acquiring new attitudes.

**Module**    A unit of academically accredited work of a stated length and worth, with its own assessment strategy.

**Pathway**    A particular combination of modules chosen from a range of optional modules within a course, which have a particular focus. Examples are the primary health care pathway and the critical care pathway.

**Personal professional portfolio**   A record of professional development, including details of relevant qualifications, continuing education activities, credits and prior and experiential learning, which may receive professional and academic recognition toward the Higher Award.

**Post-registration**   Descriptive of courses of continuing professional education and training beyond registration. The course may lead to recording of the qualification on the Professional Register.

**Pre-registration (qualifying)**   Descriptive of courses of professional preparation of nurses and midwives, leading to admission to a Part of the Professional Register.

**Shared learning**   A planned approach or strategy within curricula leading to sharing of knowledge and experience between groups.

**Supervision**   The professional support of a student by appropriately qualified staff to facilitate developing competence in the practice of nursing, midwifery or health visiting.

**Validation**   A mechanism of quality assurance, the process whereby a programme of study, its assessment and the staffing and resources available for the programme are judged to be appropriate to lead to the qualification offered.

# Appendix 2
# A Quality Guide to
# Professional Development

**1 Is the course EFFICIENT — does it achieve the desired effect with the minimum of cost?**
— Do costs compare favourably with similar programmes?
— Are there any additional costs? e.g. travel, accommodation, registration/examination fees, textbooks, VAT.
— Are there potential savings? e.g. employers may be able to recover VAT, some courses may qualify for an allowance against personal tax.
— Is the price negotiable? e.g. many training agencies will be prepared to negotiate on price to increase the number of participants on the course.
— Is the fee refundable? e.g. unavoidable absence may entitle one to a refund, deferment or substitute activity.

Comments:


**2 Is the course EFFECTIVE — does it achieve the predicted objectives/outcomes?**
— Do the course and/or its organisers have a successful record? e.g. check the views of previous participants and enquire about attrition and examination statistics.
— Is the qualification marketable? e.g. will you receive a qualification that is valued by employers, the profession and other academic institutions, or will you receive academic/vocational credit within a recognised scheme?

Comments:


**3 Is the course EQUITABLE — is it fair in its dealings?**
— Does the institution operate an equal opportunities policy? i.e. students should not be disadvantaged through race, gender, disability, pattern of study (part-time), etc.

— Are minority groups disadvantaged within a generic programme? i.e. a programme claiming to be for all nurses may still be insensitive to needs of minority groups, e.g. practice nurses, 'learning disability' nurses.

Comments:

## 4 Is the course ACCESSIBLE — free of constraint by undue limits?

— Does the programme of study fit within an academic access/accreditation scheme? e.g. credit may be given for previous learning or experience (APL/APEL) and may provide access to more advanced programmes.
— Are the institution and its facilities accessible? e.g. libraries, car parking, student union, crèche, restaurant/snack bar, facilities for the disabled.

Note: Distance learning programmes should be considered if the above factors are a problem.

Comments:

## 5 Is the course ACCEPTABLE — does it satisfy your reasonable expectations?

— Is the programme of study consistent with your learning style? e.g. despite their popularity distance learning approaches and experiential techniques are not suitable for all students.
— Is the availability of the course consistent with your professional and personal commitments?

It is worth noting that institutions and training agencies are increasingly tailoring course times to meet individual needs.

Comments:

## 6 Is the course APPROPRIATE — is it what you actually need?

This is the final and crucial consideration, the key to quality professional development.

— Is the course consistent with your personal and your organisation's needs?

An effective system of individual performance review and personal development planning should answer this question in the majority of cases.

Comments:

**Knowing your development needs**

One's own development needs are not always easy to analyse or accept. When at a career 'crossroads', for example, specialist advice may be desirable. An assessment and development centre may be well equipped to provide you with an objective appraisal of your immediate development needs.

# Index